My Klenk

Investigation of VHSV - infection models with serological methods

My Klenk

Investigation of VHSV - infection models with serological methods

Serological studies of various infection models with the viral hemorrhagic septicemia virus in rainbow trout (Oncorhynchus mykiss)

Südwestdeutscher Verlag für Hochschulschriften

Impressum/Imprint (nur für Deutschland/ only for Germany)
Bibliografische Information der Deutschen Nationalbibliothek: Die Deutsche Nationalbibliothek verzeichnet diese Publikation in der Deutschen Nationalbibliografie; detaillierte bibliografische Daten sind im Internet über http://dnb.d-nb.de abrufbar.

Alle in diesem Buch genannten Marken und Produktnamen unterliegen warenzeichen-, marken- oder patentrechtlichem Schutz bzw. sind Warenzeichen oder eingetragene Warenzeichen der jeweiligen Inhaber. Die Wiedergabe von Marken, Produktnamen, Gebrauchsnamen, Handelsnamen, Warenbezeichnungen u.s.w. in diesem Werk berechtigt auch ohne besondere Kennzeichnung nicht zu der Annahme, dass solche Namen im Sinne der Warenzeichen- und Markenschutzgesetzgebung als frei zu betrachten wären und daher von jedermann benutzt werden dürften.

Verlag: Südwestdeutscher Verlag für Hochschulschriften Aktiengesellschaft & Co. KG
Dudweiler Landstr. 99, 66123 Saarbrücken, Deutschland
Telefon +49 681 37 20 271-1, Telefax +49 681 37 20 271-0
Email: info@svh-verlag.de
Zugl.: Bern, Vetsuisse, Diss., 2008

Herstellung in Deutschland:
Schaltungsdienst Lange o.H.G., Berlin
Books on Demand GmbH, Norderstedt
Reha GmbH, Saarbrücken
Amazon Distribution GmbH, Leipzig
ISBN: 978-3-8381-1463-7

Imprint (only for USA, GB)
Bibliographic information published by the Deutsche Nationalbibliothek: The Deutsche Nationalbibliothek lists this publication in the Deutsche Nationalbibliografie; detailed bibliographic data are available in the Internet at http://dnb.d-nb.de.

Any brand names and product names mentioned in this book are subject to trademark, brand or patent protection and are trademarks or registered trademarks of their respective holders. The use of brand names, product names, common names, trade names, product descriptions etc. even without a particular marking in this works is in no way to be construed to mean that such names may be regarded as unrestricted in respect of trademark and brand protection legislation and could thus be used by anyone.

Publisher: Südwestdeutscher Verlag für Hochschulschriften Aktiengesellschaft & Co. KG
Dudweiler Landstr. 99, 66123 Saarbrücken, Germany
Phone +49 681 37 20 271-1, Fax +49 681 37 20 271-0
Email: info@svh-verlag.de

Printed in the U.S.A.
Printed in the U.K. by (see last page)
ISBN: 978-3-8381-1463-7

Copyright © 2010 by the author and Südwestdeutscher Verlag für Hochschulschriften Aktiengesellschaft & Co. KG and licensors
All rights reserved. Saarbrücken 2010

Inhaltsverzeichnis

Zusammenfassung

Serological diagnosis of several VHSV infection models of rainbow trout (*Oncorhynchus mykiss*)

Introduction	1
Materials and Methods	3
Results	14
Discussion	21
Conclusion	26
References	27
Dank	30
Methodensammlung	32

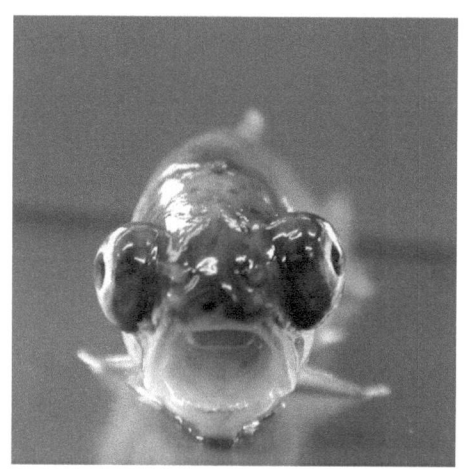

"So long and thanks for all the fish!"

(D. Adams, The Hitchhikers' Guide)

- Part I -

Serologische Studien von verschiedenen VHSV- Infektionsmodellen in Regenbogenforellen

Zusammenfassung

Die Virale Hämorrhagische Septikämie (VHS) ist eine seit langem bekannte Krankheit der Salmoniden. Diese Viruskrankheit kann grosse wirtschaftliche Verluste, besonders in Regenbogenforellen-Zuchten, verursachen. Daher ist der Erreger in der Liste der meldepflichtigen Tierseuchen der OIE (Office International de Epizooties), sowie auf der Liste II der EU Richtlinie 91/67/EEC, Annex A, sowie in der Tierseuchenverordnung der Schweiz enthalten. Als positives Resultat für das Vorhandensein der Krankheit gilt bislang der Nachweis von vermehrungsfähigem Virus. Für die Überwachung der VHS wären jedoch serologische Methoden zum Nachweis des Krankheitsstatus vorteilhaft. Serologische Nachweismethoden sind bei Säugetieren erfolgreich als indirekter Nachweis von Erkrankungen mit viralen Erregern etabliert. Bei Fischen sind bisher nur wenige serologische Tests zum Nachweis der VHS beschrieben. Das Fehlen validierter serologischer Tests für den Nachweis von VHS bei Salmoniden liegt einerseits daran, dass kaum vergleichenden Daten zu Spezifität und Sensitivität der vorhandene serologischen Methoden vorliegen, und andererseits daran, dass bisher kein reproduzierbares Modell zur Infektion von Forellen mit VHSV besteht.

Die Ziele der vorliegenden Arbeit waren eine vergleichende Untersuchung von a) verschiedenen Ansätzen zur Infektion von Regenbogenforellen mit VHSV, und b) verschiedene serologischen Methoden zum Nachweis von *anti*-VHSV-Antikörpern im Blut von Regenbogenforellen. Der Erfolg der VHSV-Behandlung wurde 5 und 10 Tage nach dessen Applikation mittels Nachweis des Virus im Fisch (virologischer Test, RT-PCR) überprüft. Es zeigte sich, dass die Manifestation des Virus mit intraperitonealer (ip.) Injektion oder in Kombination mit rektaler und ip.-Injektion am höchsten ist (>60 %). Nach rektaler Applikation war ein Virusnachweis nur in vereinzelten Fischen möglich (3 %). Eine erneute ip.-Injektion (Booster) verlief völlig symptomlos mit negativem Virusnachweis in Folge. In allen Gruppen wurde 72 Tage nach der Infektion das Serum der Fische gewonnen und die Antikörpertiter vergleichend mit einem indirekten Enzyme-linked immunosorbent Assay (ELISA), einem indirekten capture ELISA und dem Endpunkt-Seroneutralisationstest (SNT), gemessen. Die serologischen Methoden stimmten bei 70 % der untersuchten Fische überein, bei 30 % der Tiere gab es jedoch abweichende Ergebnisse. Dabei detektierte der indirekte ELISA generell weniger Positive als der capture ELISA und der SNT. Der Übereinstimmungsgrad aller serologischen Methoden war in der rektal infizierte Gruppe am höchsten (93 %), während in den Gruppen aller übrigen Applikationsarten nur eine Übereinstimmung um die 50 % ermittelt werden konnte, wobei dies sicher durch eine höhere n-Zahl noch einmal verifiziert werden müsste. Ein Effekt der Booster-Injektion durch erneute VHSV-Gabe war erkennbar, wobei sich der Unterschied eher in der Titerhöhe, als in der Anzahl seropositiver Fische zeigte. Die anhand serologischer Methoden gemessen Prävalenz von anti-VHSV-Antikörper in den verschiedenen experimentellen Gruppen zeigte nur bedingte Korrelation mit der mittels direktem Virusnachweis ermittelten Prävalenz von VHSV.

Die Ergebnisse der Arbeit zeigen, dass serologische Nachweismethoden für die VHS von Salmoniden noch methodische Weiterentwicklungen bedürfen; ein Praxiseinsatz serologischer Methoden ist damit vorläufig nicht absehbar.

Keywords: VHSV, infection models, serological methods, ELISA, SNT

Projektziele:

- Nachweis von Virus-spezifischen Antikörpern im Blut von Regenbogenforellen nach Infektion mit VHSV in Abhängigkeit von unterschiedlichen Infektionsmethoden (rektale Applikation vs. intraperitoneale Injektion; Boosterung) mit unterschiedlichen serologischen Nachweismethoden.

- Vergleich der serologischer Nachweismethoden untereinander:
    SNT (Endpunkt- Seroneutralisationstest):
    - Diese in der Agence Française de Sécurité Sanitaire des Aliments (AFSSA) Frankreich, entwickelte Methode basiert auf der Komplement-abhängigen Neutralisation der Viren durch Vorhandensein spezifischer Antikörper gegen VHSV. Dabei wird ein Fischserum-Virus-Gemisch auf eine Zellkultur aufgetragen. Der Nachweis von spezifischen Antikörpern ist dann erbracht, wenn es zur Neutralisation der Viren kommt und der Zellrasen so geschützt ist, also keine cytopathischen Effekte (CPE), ersichtlich aus Plaques, entstehen. Ein Serum ist negativ, wenn es zu einem CPE von 75-90% des Zellrasens kommt.

    ELISA (Enzyme-linked Immunosorbent Assay):
    - Die im Friedrich-Löffler-Institut (FLI), Deutschland, entwickelte Methode zum Nachweis spezifischer Antikörper gegen VHS/IHN-Viren im Fischserum basiert auf der spezifische Bindung der Antikörper an das Virus als Antigen. Das Antigen wird an ein festes Medium (ELISA-Platte) gebunden, an die wiederum die spezifischen Antikörper aus dem Serum des Fisches binden. Im Anschluss wird ein *anti*-Forellen-Antikörper aus Kaninchen aufgetragen, an dem zuletzt ein Farbstoff-markierter sekundärer *anti*-Kaninchen-Antiköper binden kann. Die Bindung dieses letzten Antiköpers an bestehende Antigen-Antikörperkomplexe führt zu einer Farbreaktion, welche gemessen werden kann.
    - Bei Anwendung der in Dänemarks Technischer Universität (DTU) in der Sektion für Fischkrankheiten entwickelten ELISA-Methode besteht der erste Schritt aus der Bindung polyklonaler Antikörper gegen das Virus an die Platte. Diese fangen im nächsten Schritt Viren aus ihrer Anzuchtlösung heraus, so dass eine Virusaufreinigung entfällt. An dem so gebundenen

Antigen können nun die spezifischen Antikörper aus dem Fischserum binden. Der weitere Aufbau gleicht der Methode des FLI. An die an das Virus gebundenen Serumantikörper aus den Fischen binden *anti*-Forellen-Antikörper aus Kaninchen. Diese werden wiederum mit Farbstoff-gebundenen *anti*-Kaninchen-Antikörpern markiert. Neben dem Unterschied im Detektionsprinzip zu der FLI-Methode wird zusätzlich jeder einzelnen Serumprobe der eigene spezifische Background durch Gegenproben ohne Virusbeschichtung abgezogen, während beim FLI Assay ein gemittelter Gruppen-Blank subtrahiert wird. Vorteil der Methode des FLI ist es, die Methode um einen Schritt zu verkürzen, Nachteil ist ein hoher Verbrauch an Virus, dessen empfindliche Aufreinigung aufwändig ist. Vorteil der Methode des DTU ist, die natürliche Bindung des Virus an der Platte durch die polyklonalen Antikörper, ohne mögliche strukturelle Verformungen. Ein Nachteil besteht darin, dass zunächst polyklonale *anti*-VHSV-Antikörper im Kaninchen hergestellt werden müssen.

- Vergleich Ergebnisse der serologischen Nachweismethoden mit etablierten Virus-Nachweismethoden (PCR, Zellkultur).

Das Projekt wurde finanziert vom schweizerischen Bundesamt für Veterinärwesen (**BVET**); Projekt.-Nr.: 1.05.07.

Introduction

Viral Haemorrhagic Septicaemia (VHS) is a well-known and one of the economically most relevant viral diseases in salmonid fish. In the middle Sixties the viral etiology was revealed by Jensen [1] and Zwillenberg [2] and today the VHS-Virus (VHSV) is classified as a *Novirhabdovirus*, part of the *Rhabdoviridae* family [3]. VHS is included in the list of notifiable diseases of the Office International de Epizooties (OIE) [4] and in List II of EU Council Directive 91/67/EEC, Annex A [5]. In Switzerland VHS is also listed as a disease to be eradicated [6]. The disease menaces mainly rainbow trout and causes annual losses of 100 Mio Euro. Therefore the surveillance of this disease is of major interest.

There are numbers of different methods to detect the VHS-virus and several of them found their way into the OIE protocols. However, one of the problems hindering eradication of VHS is, that the period for a successful diagnosis of the virus in infected fish is very short, as the virus concentration in infected fish decreases rapidly within 10 days post-infection (p.i.) [7]. In general, antibodies against a infectious agent can be detected for a longer period than the infectious agent itself. It would therefore be advantageous to have serological methods for detection of VHS infections available.

In mammals, serological methods are routinely used to detect antibodies against viruses. A major advantage of serological methods over direct virus detection is, that antibodies persist in the organism long after acute infection has ceased and the virus has disappeared from the blood or organs. Serological methods include, for instance, immunochemical tests such as Enzyme-linked Immunosorbent Assay (ELISA) or serum neutralization techniques (SNT). ELISA techniques rely on the lock-and-key-principle of antibodies and antigens, SNT methods utilize virus neutralization by antibodies, being present in the serum of the infected animals. In fish, the development and validation of serological methods for virus detection is much less progressed than in mammals. For detection of *anti*-VHSV- antibodies, only few indirect ELISAs have been described to date [8-11], but none has been validated until now. The same applies for SNTs [9-14], these tests are based on a complement dependent neutralization reaction of antibodies against VHSV. The assay is performed by using cell cultures, incubated with a mixture of complement, test serum and active virus. In comparison to the ELISA techniques, serum neutralization tests are considered to be rather specific, but less sensitive than ELISAs [10]. Overall, a gold standard for the serological detection of *anti*-VHSV-antibodies in salmonids, is not available to date.

The development and validation of serological methods for VHSV diagnosis in fish is further hindered because there is a lack of established procedures for successful and reproducible infection of salmonids with VHSV. Methods, that have been used for artificial infection of fish with VHSV include bath and oral infection, intra-peritoneal (ip.) injection or cohabitation.

Different criteria are described for the confirmation of a successful challenge infection with VHSV. The three most mentioned criteria are clinical signs of VHS, mortality and re-isolation of virus [7-9,11,15-18]. However, the correlation between the force of those criteria and the percentage of antibody induction in challenged fish does not seem to be well-defined. For instance a challenge by cohabitation caused a mortality of 70 % and a sero-prevalence of up to 32 % [10], but other reports detected much higher percentages of sero-prevalence up to 100 %, with no mortality after ip.-infection or challenge by bath [8,15,18,]. Several reports enforce booster challenge may be helpful, some show rising of antibody titers after boosting [8,11,13]. At present, there exists no standard model, for VHSV infection and induction of antibody generation in trout.

The aims of the present study are to compare: (1) the success of different techniques to infect rainbow trout with VHSV, i.e. rectal, ip., a combination of ip. and rectal, and ip. combined with an ip. booster injection - and (2) different serological methods to detect VHSV antibodies in the serum of the challenged rainbow trout. The serological tests compared in this work were: the capture ELISA of Jørgensen and Olesen [9,10], the indirect ELISA of Bergmann and Fichtner [8] and the endpoint SNT, courtesy by Jeannette Castric from the Agence Française de Securité Sanitaire des Aliments (AFSSA), Brest (France), derived from the test orriginally described by AM Hattenberger-Baudouy et al. [14]. Prevalence of infected fish per treatment were evaluated by determining a) clinical signs of disease, b) by virus isolation using the cell culture method of OIE [4], and c) by RT-PCR detection of virus RNA. A factorial experimental design was used testing all treatments with all direct virus detection methods and all serological methods.

Material and Methods

Virus

To prepare virus for the infection experiments and the serological tests we took aliquots from our frozen stock solution of the VHSV strain FI13. This strain was obtained from the National Veterinary Institute, Århus (Denmark). The thawed virus was bred on the Bluegill Fry (BF-2) cell line, cultured in Eagle's MEM with a supplement of 10 % fetal bovine serum. The cells were grown in roux-flasks (150 cm^2) for 24 h at 22°C. Virus incubation on the cells was then continued at 15°C and the cell layers were checked under an inverse microscope at least every other day for cytopathic effects (CPE). Incubation was continued until the confluent cell layer showed CPE of 70-80 %. Then, the whole medium containing virus and cells, dissolved by pipetting, was aliquoted and stored at − 80°C. Virus concentration was determined in an aliquot of the storage solution by endpoint dilution titration (s. Methodensammlung: SOP_smv018). Afterwards, the virus concentration was calculated according to Spearman-Kaerber formula (s. Methodensammlung: SOP_smv018) [19] as tissue culture infective doses, giving 50% effect (TCID$_{50}$). For this VHSV stock solution (VHSV70%), the calculated concentration was 1.3×10^9 TCID$_{50}$. The VHSV70% was taken for the infection experiments in a final concentration of 1.3×10^5 TCID$_{50}$/ml, diluted in phosphate-buffered-saline (PBS: 0.14 M NaCl; 2.7 mM KCl; 4.6 mM Na$_2$HPO$_4$.2H$_2$O; 1.8 mM KH$_2$PO$_4$; adjusted with 1 M NaOH to pH 7.4). Undiluted aliquots of the VHSV70% stock solution were also used for the capture ELISA.

For the indirect ELISA, another virus stock was prepared. Virus was inoculated as described above, but the incubation was not stopped until the CPE reached 100 %. The resulting VHSV stock solution (VHSV100%) was used for virus purification. For purification (s. Methodensammlung), gross cell detritus was separated by several centrifugation steps using the centrifuges Centrikon T-124 and Centrikon T-2070 (Kontron Instruments, Groß-Zimmern, Germany), from the VHSV100% stock solution, followed by ultra-centrifugation with the Centrikon T-2070 (s.a.) on a saccharose gradient (20 %, 40 %, 50 %, 60 %). After ultra centrifugation, bands of virus particles at the 40 % and 50 % saccharose layer were picked and pelleted by an additional ultra-centrifugation step. The concentration of the purified virus

(VHSVpurif) was measured using the NanoDrop photometer (s.a.) and diluted with TNE-Puffer (0.02M TRIS; 0.1M NaCl; 0.005M EDTA; pH 8.6) to a final concentration of 1 mg/ml. Then, the purified virus solution was divided in aliquots of 33 µl and stored at − 80°C until usage.

Positive and negative control sera

A total of 20 rainbow trout, survivors from an infection experiment, performed in the FIWI facilities, were used for producing a positive control serum for the following serological tests. The fish were originally obtained from a farm, which has a history of being free of VHSV and IHNV since more than 25 years (regular controls twice per year). Fish were of 2+ age and had a size of 30-35 cm. The fish received in the first infection experiment 0.05 ml of the VHSV70% diluted in PBS to a concentration of 1.3×10^2 $KCID_{50}$/ml by rectal application. Then, 14 month later, four further injections in intervals of 4 weeks. The fish were challenged again by rectal application of 100 µl diluted VHSV70% stock solution. This time, for the initial booster a dilution of VHSV70% with PBS (1:100.000), resulting in 1.3×10^4 was used. For the following booster injections the virus concentration was increased at each injection by one order of magnitude until the highest concentration of 1.3×10^7 $KCID_{50}$/ml. For sampling of the sera, 4 weeks after last booster, fish were anesthetized with MS 222 (Triacin-Methansulfonat) and blood was sampled by puncture of caudal vein. To divide serum from cells, the blood was centrifuged at 4°C and 3000g for 5 min, aliquoted and then stored at − 80°C. As negative controls, sera were taken from fish of the same farm as described above. These latter fish had a size of 35-38 cm and were aged 1+.

All positive and negative sera were tested with the indirect ELISA (s.b.) to ascertain that they were positive and negative, respectively. Only the best positive and negative serum was taken for the measurements. Their functionality was affirmed by the other serological tests before starting measurement with each method, as well.

Experimental design

A total of 360 rainbow trout (*Oncorhynchus mykiss*) were obtained from a farm, which is tested negative for VHS since 20 years (regularly tested twice per year). Fish (0+), measured about 90 mm and weighed about 9 g. They were divided into six groups (B9-B14) and kept in glass aquaria with a flow-through of approximately 0,6 l/min of tap water. The fish were fed commercial trout pellets (Hokovit Silver Cup, Bützberg, Switzerland). After transfer from the farm, fish were acclimated to the laboratory conditions for seven days before starting the infection experiments.

As a specificity control, one of the experimental groups (B9) was challenged with a non-viral agent: *Yersinia (Y.) ruckeri*, strain JF 3685. Yersinia is known to induce a strong humoral response in fish; thus, this pathogen was used to evaluate whether the ELISA response is specific to VHSV antibodies or shows unspecific bindings of other antibodies [11]. The bacteria were cultivated in Luria – Bertoni (LB) medium at 25°C overnight. Cell number was determined spectrophotometrically and verified by plate counting in colony forming units (cfu) for the final working dilution of 5×10^5 cfu/ml with PBS for the infection.

For infecting the fish with the pathogens, they were anesthetized with MS 222 and injected according to the infection scheme below (Tab.1). The two groups B10 and B11 were ip.- challenged with 0.05 ml per fish of the VHSV challenge solution (s.a.: 1.3×10^5 TCID$_{50}$/ml). The group B10 received 25 days after the initial infection a second injection with the same concentration of VHSV (booster injection). The group B12 was challenged by a combination of 0.025 ml ip.-injection and 0.025 ml rectal-injection per fish. Finally, the group B13 was injected only rectally (rect.) with 0.05 ml VHSV challenge solution per fish. Two control groups were used: group B14 as negative control in which each fish was ip.-injected with 0.05 ml PBS and group B9, as a specificity control, receiving 0.05 ml of the *Y. ruckeri* solution (s.a.) per fish by intra-peritoneal challenge. As baseline samples for serology and virus isolation, sera and organs from ten fish were taken, immediately before the beginning of experiment (day 0).

Fore collecting sera at day 72 post-infection (pi.), fish were euthanized with an overdose of MS 222. Blood samples from individual fish were obtained by puncture of the caudal vein. The blood was centrifuged at 4°C, 3000 g, for 5 min to separate serum from blood cells. After aliquoting the sera, they were stored at - 80°C until examination.

In addition to the sera, also tissue samples for virus detection were collected on days 5 and 10 post-infection. At each sampling, organ pieces were taken from 15 fish per group, except B9 (Y. ruckeri), where only 10 and 9 fish could be sampled due to the high mortality in this group. Of each individual fish two equal subsamples consisting of organ pieces from heart, kidney, spleen and liver were collected. One subsample was stored in a tube with 1 ml RNAlater® Soln. (Ambion, Forster City, CA, USA) for RT-PCR and the second aliquot was stored in a tube with 1 ml antibiotic solution (s. Methodensammlung: SOP_smv003) for virus re-isolation on cell culture.

Table 1: Infection scheme and overview of sampling time points during the experiment.

	Y. ruckeri	VHSV				PBS	
day	B9 ip.	B10 ip. boost.	B11 ip.	B12 ip. + rect.	B13 rect.	B14 ip.	samples
0	2	2	2	2	2	2	organs, sera
5	10	15	15	15	15	15	organs
10	9	15	15	15	15	15	organs
72	remaining	remaining	remaining	remaining	remaining	remaining	sera

boost.: boosted; ip.: intraperitoneal; rect.: rectal; Y.: Yersinia; remaining: sampling of remaining fish after 72 days post-infection

Virological analysis

Virus incubation in cell culture

For the detection of virus in infected fish the method described in Annex, Part III of the Commission Decision of the European Communities [5] was applied with some modifications as described in Knüsel et al. [12]. Briefly, cells of a BF-2 cell line, preferred by VHSV, were seeded in 48-well plates in Eagle's MEM with a supplement of 10 % fetal bovine serum and were grown for 24 h at 22°C. Homogenized organ material from individual fish was centrifuged (4°C, 2000 g, 20 min) and 100 µl of the upper layer of the supernatant, diluted 1:10 in PBS, were inoculated onto the cell cultures. The cells were then incubated at 15°C and checked at least every other day for CPE under an inverse microscope. If CPE developed, the virus was identified by

Indirect Fluorescence Antibody Technique (IFAT). If no CPE developed after 7 days of incubation, 100 µl of supernatant from each well was transferred into a fresh cell culture well and incubated for another 7-day-period. If there was still no CPE seen, the sample was considered to be negative.

IFAT (Indirect Fluorescent Antibody Technique)

To identify virus grown on cell cultures, we applied the IFAT following the protocol delivered with the BIO-FLUO-kit (Bio-X, Marcheen-Famenne, Belgium) for VHSV. Modifications are described in detail by Knüsel et al. [12]. Cells from all wells of a particular sample showing CPE were scraped off and pooled after discharging most of supernatant. One drop of the pooled cells was pipetted into six wells of a defatted slide holder glass (Standard 25 mm x 75 mm immunofluorescent printed slides, with 12x5 mm-wells, Semadeni AG, Ostermundingen, Switzerland). Drying (2-4 h) at room temperature (rt) was followed by fixation with 100% isopropanol (40-60 min) and a further drying (15 min, rt). Then the probes were stored at - 20°C until further processing. As positive controls, slides containing VHSV infected cells were used.
After thawing, slides with the fixed cells were washed (10 min, PBS) and dried again (15 min). 10 µl of the VHS-antiserum were pipetted into two wells (no antiserum was pipetted into the wells with the negative controls). On the slides with the positive controls two wells were overlaid with the VHSV-antiserum and two further wells were covered with anti-IHNV serum, as a non-corresponding antiserum control. The monoclonal antibodies were obtained from two different sources: 1) Commercial kits: BIO-FLUO-kit for VHS (s.a.); 2) a Rabbit anti VHS-virus antiserum (DK rabbit F38) kindly provided from the National Veterinary Institute, Århus (Denmark). The slides were incubated with 10 µl of the monoclonal antibody solutions for 2 h at room temperature (rt) in a humid chamber before washing (10 min, PBS) and drying (15 min, rt). Ten µl of fluorescein isothiocyanate-conjugated *anti*-mouse antiserum (BIO-FLUO-kit) or a swine *anti*-rabbit-IgG (Dako, Zug, Switzerland) antiserum for the Danish antibodies, respectively, were added. Slides were then incubated in a humid chamber (1 h, rt), washed (10 min, distilled water), covered with mounting medium (BIO-FLUO-Kits) and stored (humid chamber, 4°C) for a maximum of 2 h until reading.

Reading the slides was done in a fluorescence microscope. The results were considered as positive if fluorescence was observed in the samples with the specific antibodies, and if these samples showed no reaction with antibodies against other viruses (s. non-corresponding antiserum). In case of questionable results the procedure was repeated.

RT-PCR (Reverse Transcriptase- Polymerase Chain Reaction)

A method based on a protocol described by Bergmann, Olesen, Frank Skall, Einer-Jensen and Fichtner [20] was used with some modifications according to Knüsel at al. [21]. Total RNA was extracted by using TRIzol-Reagent® (Invitrogen, Basel, Switzerland) according to the instructions of the manufacturers. The RNA was eluted in 50 to 100 µl RNA-Storage Solution® (Ambion Inc., Austin, Texas, USA). The quality and quantity of the purified RNA was determined by measuring the absorbance at 260 nm (A_{260}) and 280 nm (A_{280}) in a NanoDrop photometer (NanoDrop Technologies, Inc., Wilmington, USA). In the subsequent one-step RT-PCR 1µl (50 pmol/µl) of each forward and reverse primer, and 1µg of template-RNA were added to the "mastermix" (Quiagen OneStep® RT-PCR-Kit, Quiagen, Basel, Switzerland) to give a final volume of 50 µl. As primer sequences, those published by Knüsel et al. [11] were used. The thermocycler (PTC-200 DNA Engine, MJ Research, BioConcept, Allschwil, Switzerland) was programmed as follows: 1:50°C for 40 min (reverse transcription); 2: 95°C for 15 min followed by 35 cycles (with additional 5 sec per cycle) at 94°C for 1 min; 52°C for 1 min; 72°C for 1 min and final extension at 72°C for 10 min.

Six µl of the RT-PCR products were electrophoresed at 100 volts for 1 hour on a 1.5% agarose-TAE (TRIS-acetat, EDTA, pH 8.0) gel. The gel was then stained with SYBR® Green I nucleic acid gel stain (Molecular Probes, Eugene, Oregon, USA) and the bands were visualized in a transilluminator Tm-36 (Ultra Violet Products Ltd., Cambridge, UK).

Serological analyses

SNT (end point Seroneutralization Test)

The protocol of the endpoint seroneutralization test is derived from the one described by AM Hattenberger-Baudouy et al. [14] and was kindly performed by Jeannette Castric from the Agence Française de Sécurité Sanitaire des Aliments (AFFSA), Brest, France. Before starting measurements with the SNT, the reference virus used for the SNT had to be titrated. This reference VHSV strain was the isolate 07/71, genotype I-a [31] from diseased rainbow trout. The virus stock, grown on Epithelioma Papulosum Cyprini (EPC) cells in cell culture medium (s.b.) and used for SNT, was aliquoted to 0.5 ml and kept at − 80°C. An aliquot of the virus was thawed for virus endpoint dilution titration in 96-wells microplates containing EPC cells in culture medium: Glasgow Minimum Essential medium (Sigma-Aldrich Corporation, St. Luis, MO, USA), buffered at pH 7.6 with TRIS-HCL (0.19M), supplemented with 10 % tryptose phosphate broth, 10 % foetal bovine serum and standard antibiotic solution of penicillin (10^6 International Units [IU]/l) and streptomycin (1g/l). At the end of the titration, the cells were fixed and stained using crystal violet solution (1.3 g crystal violet powder, dissolved in 100 ml ethanol and 400 ml distilled water) and the infectious titer was determined as $TCID_{50}$ by using the Kaerber formula (s. Methodensammlung: SOP_smv018) [19].

For the SNT, 150 µl of an EPC cell suspension (20×10^4 cells/well) per well were seeded into flat bottom wells of 96-well microplates. Cells were incubated at 29°C for 24-48 h. Twin plates were prepared for each serie of sera and for the controls. Two plates were used for 20 sera diluted from 1:40 to 1:320 plus the two twin plates for the control.

The sera to be tested were de-complemented by heat treatment at 45°C for 30 min. Pre-dilutions of 1:20 (20 µl Serum and 380 µl medium) were diluted in tubes and were maintained at 3-5°C until end of the analysis, so that in case of problems, those tubes could be used to perform the test again. Afterwards, a geometrical dilution serie of each serum was given into round bottom 96-wells microplates.

For each plate, 3 ml of the viral suspension of the reference strain VHSV 07/71, containing 6×10^4 $TCID_{50}$, were diluted in cell culture medium containing complement (s. Methodensammlung: SOP_msv008) at a final dilution of 1:20. Then, 30 µl of the viral suspension (about 600 $TCID_{50}$) was added in each well of the plates containing the serum solutions to be tested, beginning with the highest dilution. Viral suspension was added to the control plates as well.

On the twin control plates, the different control mixtures were prepared as follows:
1) pure cell culture medium
2) 1:1 cell culture medium and medium containing complement, used for virus dilution
3) 1:1 cell culture medium and viral suspension (s.a.), containing complement
4) 1:1 each dilution of a negative *anti*-VHSV serum and virus suspension
5) 1:1 each dilution (1:80 to 1:10240 or more) of a standard *anti*-VHSV serum of known titer plus virus suspension

Afterwards the plates were shaken gently for about 5 min and then incubated for 16 h to 24 h at 3-5°C. Then, transfer of 50 µl of all dilutions to the corresponding wells of the plates containing EPC cells took place, again beginning with the highest dilution of the sera until the lowest. The plates containing EPC cells and inoculated with the serum-virus mixtures and control dilutions were incubated at 14°C during 3 to 4 days. After three days incubation, microscopical examination of the plates was done. The following criteria had to be fulfilled: a) the cells of the controls had to be intact; b) the cell sheet in the standard virus control had to be destroyed at 75 to 90% compared to the cell control and c) the standard positive serum had a neutralizing titer of 5120. If those conditions were met, the plates were fixed and stained by discarding the medium and staining with 50 µl of crystal violet solution per well for at least 1 h. Then the colorant was discarded, the plates were rinsed the plates with tap water until the color of the water turned pale purple and afterwards the plates were left for drying at rt.

For reading and interpretation the test results, the following conditions had to be met in order to get interpretable results: 1) cell controls showed a correct cell layer with and without complement; 2) incubation with the control virus had to cause 75 - 90% destruction of the cell layer; 3) control negative serum had to show the same intensity of cell layer destruction as the standard virus control; 4) The standard positive serum yielded neutralizing titer of 5120. The neutralizing titer was the inverse of the serum dilution, giving the 50% neutralization of the reference VHSV compared to the virus control on the control plate. All sera with a neutralizing titer equal or higher than 80 were considered as positive. No statistic program was used, this threshold is derived from historical data. As negative and positive serum controls, in-house sera were taken, but also our positive and negative control sera were affirmed as correct highly positive and negative.

ELISA (Enzyme Linked Immune Sorbent Assay)

Indirect capture ELISA

For detecting anti-VHSV antibodies in rainbow trout with the indirect capture ELISA, we followed the previously described technique of Jørgensen and Olesen [9,10]. As first layer, the wells of 96-well microtiter plates (Greiner) were coated with Protein-A purified rabbit anti-VHSV immunoglobulin (Ig), produced at the National Veterinary Institute [3]. For coating, the anti-VHSV Ig was diluted 1:750 in bicarbonate buffer (7,5 mM Na_2CO_3; 17,44 mM $NaHCO_3$; pH 9,6). Per well, 50 µl of the anti-VHSV immunoglobulin (Ig) solution were added and incubated overnight at 4°C on an orbital shaker. After washing three times with PBS (2.5 mM $NaH_2PO_4.H_2O$; 7.5 mM $Na_2HPO_4.12H_2O$; 0.15 M NaCl; setting up with 1 M NaOH to pH 7.4) containing 0.05% Tween-20 (PBS-T), the plates were incubated with 50 µl virus dilution, containing VHSV70% stock solution (s. Virus), diluted 1:10 in PBS-T with 1 % bovine serum albumin (PBS-T-BSA), for 1 h at rt on an orbital shaker. After washing with PBS-T, plates were blocked with 100 µl PBS-T-BSA per well for 2 h at rt. Then, after another washing with PBS-T, plates were incubated with fish sera in serial 4-fold dilution steps (1:40 to 1:2560). The sera dilutions were added to wells, either with and without virus. All sera were tested in duplicates. Plates with serum solutions were incubated overnight at 4°C on an orbital shaker. After washing, 50 µl of a mixture of two monoclonal antibodies against rainbow trout IgM Monoclonal antibodies (Mab) 4C10 diluted at 1:50, and Mab D_2, diluted at 1:100 in PBS-T per well. Both antibodies were kindly provided by the National Veterinary Institute, Århus (Denmark) [22]. Incubation was done for 1 h at rt on an orbital shaker. Following another washing step with PBS-T, the plates were incubated with HRP (horseradish peroxidase) conjugated rabbit Ig against mouse Ig, followed by a final washing step. The bound enzyme was visualized by adding 50 µl of H_2O_2-σ-phenylenediamine(OPD)-substrate solution (0.4mg/ml OPD-tablet (Sigma-Aldrich Corporation, St. Luis, MO, USA), activated with 4 µl 30 % H_2O_2, in 10 ml phosphate-citrate-buffer [phosphate: 0,2M dibasic sodium phosphate; citrate: 0,1M citric acid; pH 5.0]) to each well. Enzyme activity was stopped after 10-20 min with 50 µl of 4N H_2SO_4 acid and the absorbance was recorded at 492 nm (A_{492}), using a Titertek Multisscan reader.

The analysis followed exactly to the protocol of Olesen and Jørgensen [9,10]. In this ELISA, antigen was first captured by polyclonal rabbit anti-VHSV antibodies, so that purification of virus was not necessary. Because of the distinct tendency of fish antibodies to non-specific binding on the plates, each fish serum acted as its own negative control by incubating the sera on wells with and without virus, and calculating the background-corrected optical density value from the difference between the two wells. The ELISA titer was defined as a reciprocal value of the highest serum dilution giving a difference in absorbance of 0.5 or more between wells with and without virus, respectively. Titers were categorized into in five dilution levels: <40, 40, 160, 640 and 2560. On each plate, negative and positive control sera (s.a.) were included.

Indirect ELISA

The indirect ELISA was developed by Bergmann and Fichtner [8]. The VHSVpurif (s.a.) was diluted in bicarbonate buffer to an end concentration of 3.3 µg/ml. Then, 100 µl of this virus solution was filled in the wells of a 96-wells microplate (Polysorb Nunc F), according to scheme (s. Methodensammlung). The plates were incubated in a humid chamber overnight at 4°C. Then, the plates were washed three times with PBS (s. capture ELISA) containing 0.05 % Tween 20 (PBS-T) and blocked with 200 µl Roti-Block (Roth, Germany) reagent (10 %) per well for 1h at rt. After washing three times with PBS, serial dilutions of fish sera were added to the wells starting with 1:50 up to 1:1600, according to the scheme (s. Methodensammlung). Each sample was added in duplicate. Plates were incubated for 1h at rt and washed again three times. Afterwards, 100 µl of an *anti*-rainbow-trout-IgM Mab (s. Mab 4C10 capture ELISA) dilution (1:200 in PBS-T), were given in each well and incubated for 1h at rt. After washing three times, 100 µl of the *Anti*-Mouse IgG-Peroxidase (produced in rabbit; Sigma-Aldrich Corporation, St. Luis, MO, USA), diluted in PBS-T (1:5000), were added in each well and incubated for 1h at rt. Then, after another three times washing, 100 µl of a H_2O_2-OPD-substrate solution (s. indirect capture ELISA) were added to each well. Enzyme activity was stopped after 10-20 min with 50 µl of 4 N H_2SO_4 acid and the absorbance was recorded at 492 nm (A_{492}) using the Wallac Victor^2 1420 Multilabel Counter (PerkinElmer, Salem, MA, USA). As controls, the negative and positive control sera described above were added on each plate. Due to the incubation scheme (s. Methodensammlung), all marginal wells of the plates were provided as blanks. The absorbance of the mean blank on each plate was calculated and divided from each tested serum OD.

The threshold of absorbance was estimated on the basis of mean values of negative control sera. Values were tested for normality and analyzed using ANOVA on ranks. Results were considered significantly different with p<0.05. All statistical analysis were performed with NCSS [23]. According to the protocol of Bergmann and Fichtner [8], values less than 200 were regarded as negatives, that also agreed to our calculations (s. Results).

Results

Clinical and virological examination

About one week post-infection (pi.) first clinical signs in groups B10-B13 were observed in some of the infected fish. The time point of clinical disease manifestation varied slightly between the treatments, with group B12 (ip. + rect.), being the first one showing diseased fish, followed by the groups B10 and B11, both receiving ip.-injections, and with the group B13 (rect.) being the last one. The clinical signs included external characteristics like dark skin, pale gills, exophthalmos and anemia as well as internal lesions like comma-formed bleedings in skeletal muscle, petechial to blotty bleedings in ocular connective tissue and viscera, swollen kidneys and pale liver were found. All these signs are described to be typical for an acute VHS infection [24]. Fish from group B9 displayed typical symptoms of a bacterial septicemia and high mortality since 3 days post-infection (Tab.2). Signs like dark skin, exophthalmos, ascites, bleedings over abdominal organs, swollen and reddened kidney and spleen [24] were observed. By taking a smear of dead fish for cultivation on blood agar plates and afterwards, the grown bacteria were identified as *Y. ruckeri* by Bunte series.

Cumulative mortality (Tab.2) during the experimental period was highest in B12 (ip. + rect.), although the amount of administered virus was identical in all groups (s. Material and Methods). In the group B10 (ip. boosted), mortality was marginally different to groups B11 and B13 (Tab.2), even after the second ip. treatment. Thus, all VHSV-infected groups showed an almost identical low mortality (6-9 %), except B12. Dead fish were checked for clinical signs and tested VHSV-positive by virus re-isolation. In the control group B14 (PBS ip.), two fish died, but this was due to a bacteraemia caused by an agent different to *Y. ruckeri*. Probably this infection resulted from the injection treatment. In group B9, where fish had been injected Y. ruckeri, total mortality reached 50 %.

Table 2: Mortalities during the first four weeks p.i. and results of the VHSV re-isolation (re-isol.) from the dead fish.

	Y. ruckeri	VHSV				PBS
	B9	B10	B11	B12	B13	B14
week	ip.	ip. boosted	ip.	ip. + rect.	rect.	ip.
1	12			1		
2	6	4	2	14	2	
3			1	2		2
4		1			3	
total	28	5	3	17	5	2
% mortality	50	9	6	27	9	4

B9: infected with Y. ruckeri, B10-13: infected with VHSV, B14: injected with PBS; boost.: boosted at day 25 post-infection; ip.: intraperitoneal; rect.: rectal

At days 5 and 10 after infection, organ samples were taken from 15 alive fish out of each group and were tested for the presence of virus by means of virus re-isolation and RT-PCR (Tabs.3,4). Prevalence of virus-positive fish differed markedly between the groups. The highest prevalence were observed in the groups B11 (ip.) and B12 (ip.+rect.), while the lowest prevalence was found in the group B13 (rect.). Overall, in all groups RT-PCR detected more virus-positive samples than virus re-isolation. Both for day 5 and day 10 post-infection, RT-PCR detected the highest number of virus-positive fish in group B12 (ip.+ rect.). Group B11 - one of the ip.-injected groups - had slightly lower numbers of virus-positive fish than B12. The other ip.- injected group B10 had a much lower prevalence virus-positives fish than group B11. Therefore we had chosen this group for the second (booster) infection (B10: ip. boosted). Clearly the lowest number of fish, that were tested positive for the virus by RT-PCR, were present in group B13 (rect.). Both, RT-PCR and virus re-isolation revealed negative results for fish of the *Y. ruckeri* infected group B9 and for fish of the PBS injected group B14. Samples taken from fish before infection (baseline; day 0), were all tested negative for the presence of VHSV (data not shown) with RT-PCR and virus re-isolation.

Table 3: Detection of VHSV infection of fish either by means of the virus re-isolation (re-isol.) or by means of RT-PCR. Samples were taken at day 5 post-infection. 1= positive; 0= negative

fish	B9 ip.		B10 ip. boost.		B11 ip.		B12 ip. + rect.		B13 rect.		B14 ip.	
	re-isol.	PCR	re-isol.	PCR	re-isol.	PCR	re-isol.	PCR	re-isol.	PCR	re-isol.	PCR
1	0	0	0	1	0	0	0	0	0	0	0	0
2	0	0	0	0	0	0	1	1	0	0	0	0
3	0	0	0	0	0	0	0	1	0	0	0	0
4	0	0	0	0	1	1	1	1	0	0	0	0
5	0	0	0	1	1	1	0	0	0	0	0	0
6	0	0	0	0	1	1	1	1	0	0	0	0
7	0	0	1	1	1	1	0	0	0	0	0	0
8	0	0	0	0	0	0	0	0	0	0	0	0
9	0	0	1	1	0	1	0	1	0	0	0	0
10	0	0	0	1	1	1	1	1	0	0	0	0
11			0	1	0	0	0	1	0	0	0	0
12			0	0	1	1	0	0	0	0	0	0
13			1	1	0	1	1	1	0	0	0	0
14			0	0	1	1	0	0	0	0	0	0
15			0	0	1	1	0	1	0	0	0	0
sub.	*0*	*0*	*3*	*7*	*8*	*10*	*5*	*9*	*0*	*0*	*0*	*0*
			20%	46.60%	53.30%	66.60%	33.30%	60%	0			

B9: infected with Y. ruckeri, B10-13: infected with VHSV, B14: injected with PBS; boost.: boosted (at day 25 post-indection); ip.: intraperitoneal; rect.: rectal

Table 4: Detection of VHSV infection of fish with either by means of the virus re-isolation (re-isol.) or by means of RT-PCR. Samples were taken at day 10 post-infection. 1= positive; 0= negative

Fish	B9 ip.		B10 ip. boost.		B11 ip.		B12 ip. + rect.		B13 rect.		B14 ip.	
	re-isol.	PCR	re-isol.	PCR	re-isol.	PCR	re-isol.	PCR	re-isol.	PCR	re-isol.	PCR
1	0	0	0	0	0	0	1	1	0	0	0	0
2	0	0	0	0	1	1	0	0	0	0	0	0
3	0	0	1	1	0	1	0	0	0	0	0	0
4	0	0	0	0	0	0	1	1	1	1	0	0
5	0	0	1	1	1	1	1	1	0	0	0	0
6	0	0	0	0	1	1	0	0	0	0	0	0
7	0	0	0	0	1	1	1	1	0	0	0	0
8	0	0	0	0	1	1	1	1	0	0	0	0
9	0	0	0	0	1	1	1	1	0	0	0	0
10			1	1	0	0	0	0	0	0	0	0
11			0	1	0	0	0	0	0	0	0	0
12			0	0	0	0	0	1	0	0	0	0
13			0	1	1	1	1	1	0	0	0	0
14			0	0	0	0	0	1	0	0	0	0
15			0	0	0	0	0	1	0	0	0	0
sub.	*0*	*0*	*3*	*5*	*7*	*8*	*7*	*10*	*1*	*1*	*0*	*0*
			20%	33.30%	46.60%	53.30%	46.60%	66.60%	6.60%	6.60%		

| total | *0* | *0* | *6* | *12* | *15* | *18* | *12* | *19* | *2* | *1* | *0* | *0* |
| | | | 20% | 40% | 50% | 60% | 40% | 63.30% | 3.30% | 3.30% | | |

B9: infected with Y. ruckeri, B10-13: infected with VHSV, B14: injected with PBS; boost.: boosted (at day 25 post-infection); ip.: intraperitoneal; rect.: rectal; sub.: subtotal; total: combined results from samples take at day 5 and day 10 post-infection

Serological analysis of anti VHSV antibodies was done on fish sampled at day 72 after infection. Serum was taken from fish after euthanization. All three serological techniques detected antibodies in fish from the VHSV-treated groups, but were negative - with one exception (s. Tab.6+7) - for the negative control as well as for the group challenged with *Y. ruckeri*, that confirming the specificity of the methods. The number of fishes tested sero-positive for VHSV-antibodies varied between the experimental groups, but also between the three tested serological methods.

The indirect ELISA (Tab.5) provides a semi-quantitative estimate of antibody titers, which were defined as a reciprocal value of the highest serum dilution giving a difference in absorbance of 0.095 or more between the serum to test and the mean blank of the ELISA-plate (s. Materials and Methods). According to the protocol of Bergmann and Fichtner [8], that also agreed to our calculations, values less than 200 were regarded as negatives. With the indirect ELISA, the highest percentage of fish sera containing VHSV antibodies was found in the group B10 (ip. boosted).

Table 5: Results of the indirect ELISA for the detection of *anti*-VHSV-antibodies in serum of infected rainbow trout. Blood was sampled at day 72 post-infection.
Reciprocal dilutions were calculated as mean values. Numbers in **bold** depict fish with positive antibody titers. Values less than 200 were regarded as negative.

fish	B9 ip.	B10 ip. boost.	B11 i.p.	B12 ip.+rect.	B13 rect.	B14 ip.	baseline
1	100	**400**	**800**	100	50	50	<50
2	50	**200**	50		**200**	100	50
3	50	**200**	100	**200**	50	50	<50
4	<50	100	**200**	<50	50	50	<50
5	<50	**200**	50	100	**800**	<50	50
6	50	**400**	100	**200**	<50	50	<50
7	<50	50	100	<50	<50	50	<50
8	<50	50	100	100	<50	<50	<50
9	<50	**400**	50	50	<50	<50	50
10		100	50	<50	50	<50	<50
11		**200**	**>1600**	50	<50	<50	
12		50	**>1600**	<50	**400**	<50	
13		**>1600**	<50	<50	100	<50	
14		**800**	50	<50	<50	<50	
15		**200**	100	<50	<50	<50	
16		**800**	**400**	**200**	**>1600**	<50	
17		**200**	**400**		100		
		100			<50		
		>1600			<50		
		50			50		
		13/20	6/16	3/15	4/20		
		65%	38%	20%	20%		

B9: infected with Y. ruckeri, B10-13: infected with VHSV, B14: injected with PBS; baseline: sera, briefly taken before challenge; boost.: boosted at day 25 p.i.; ip.: intraperitoneal; rect.: rectal

The sera of 13 out of 20 fish reacted positive in the indirect ELISA. Values in the groups receiving only a single administration of virus were clearly lower than in the boosted group. The percentage of sero-positive fish ranged between 38 % sero-positives in group 11 (ip.) and 20 % in both groups B12 (ip.+rect.) and B13 (rect.). All sera of the control groups B9 (Y. ruckeri), B14 (PBS ip.) and the baseline group were tested negative for *anti*-VHSV antibodies with the indirect ELISA.

The same sera tested in the indirect ELISA were also assayed in the indirect capture ELISA (Tab.6). This assay also provides a semi-quantitative estimate of antibody titers, which were defined as a reciprocal value of the highest serum dilution giving a difference in absorbance of 0.5 or more between the wells containing sera and coated with and without virus (s. Materials and Methods). According to the protocol of Olesen and Jørgensen [9,10], values less than 160 were regarded as negatives. Measurements with the capture ELISA revealed a clear ranking, starting with group B10 (ip. boosted) with 80 % positive sera. Then, 71 % positives in the single challenged group B11 (ip.), followed by group B12 (ip.+ rect.) with 53 % and finally group B13 (rect.) with 36 % positive sera.

Table 6: Results of the indirect capture ELISA for the detection of *anti*-VHSV-antibodies in serum of infected rainbow trout. Blood was sampled at day 72 post-infection.
Reciprocal dilutions were calculated as mean values. Numbers in **bold** depict fish with positive antibody titers. Values less than 160 were regarded as negative.

fish	B9 ip.	B10 ip. boost.	B11 ip.	B12 ip.+rect.	B13 rect.	B14 ip.	baseline
1	<40		>2560	<40	<40	<40	<40
2	<40	160	<40	<40	640	<40	<40
3	<40	>2560	640	640	<40	640	<40
4	<40	>2560	640	<40	<40	<40	<40
5	<40	>2560	40	<40	>2560	<40	<40
6	<40	>2560	<40	640	160	<40	<40
7	<40	<40	640	40	640	<40	<40
8	<40	640	640	>2560	<40	<40	<40
9	<40	>2560	640	>2560		<40	<40
10		640	160	640	40	<40	<40
11		>2560	>2560	160	<40	<40	
12		40	>2560	40	>2560	<40	
13		>2560	<40	640	<40	<40	
14		640	<40	>2560	<40	<40	
15			640	<40	<40	<40	
16		>2560	>2560				
17		40	640				
		12/15	12/17	8/15	5/14	1/15	
		80%	71%	53%	36%	7%	

B9: infected with Y. ruckeri, B10-13: infected with VHSV, B14: injected with PBS; baseline: sera, briefly taken before challenge; boost.: boosted; ip.: intraperitoneal; rect.: rectal

The sera of the control groups B9 and the baseline were tested negative for anti-VHSV antibodies with the capture ELISA. In one fish of the control group B14 (PBS ip.) a positive titer was found.

Finally, all sera were tested in the SNT (Tab.7). The SNT is a semi-quantitative test as well. Four dilution levels were analyzed for the presence of anti-VHSV antibodies. According to the protocol of the AFSSA, titers were determines as the reciprocal value of the highest serum dilution of test serum, showing 50 % neutralization of the reference VHSV compared to the virus control well giving 75-90 % CPE (s. Materials and Methods). Values less than 80 were regarded as negatives. For the groups that received a single VHSV application, the SNT yielded a ranking in the prevalence of sero-positive fish from, group B11 (ip.), followed by group B12 (ip. + rect.) and finally group B13 (rect.). The group B10 (ip. boosted) showed no clearly difference to the single challenged group B11 (ip.) in numbers of sero-positives, but as in the other serological methods the SNT detected higher titers in this group compared to the single challenged groups.

Table 7: Results of the SNT for the detection of anti-VHSV-antibodies in serum of infected rainbow trout. Blood was sampled at day 72 post-infection.
Reciprocal dilutions were calculated as mean values. Numbers in **bold** depict fish with positive antibody titers. Values less than 80 were regarded as negative. - = negative response

fish	B9 ip.	B10 ip. boost.	B11 ip.	B12 ip.+rect.	B13 rect.	B14 ip.	baseline
1	-		>320		-	-	-
2	-	>320	-		>320	-	-
3	-	160	80		-	-	-
4	-	-	-	-	-	-	-
5	-	>320	80	320	320	-	-
6	-	>320	-	>320	-	-	-
7	-	-	80	-	-	-	-
8	-	-	80	160	-	-	-
9	-	>320	>320	<320		-	-
10		160/320	>320		-	-	-
11		-	>320	>320	-	-	
12		320	160	>320	320	320	
13		>320	-	-	-	-	
14		160	40		-	-	
15			320		-	-	
16		>320	>320				
17		-	>320				
		10/14	12/17	6/9	3/14	1/15	
		71%	76%	67%	21%	7%	

B9: infected with Y. ruckeri, B10-13: infected with VHSV, B14: injected with PBS; baseline: sera, briefly taken before challenge; boost.: boosted; ip.: intraperitoneal; rect.: rectal

All sera from control groups B9 and the baseline tested negative for *anti*-VHSV antibodies with the SNT, but in one serum out of the group B14 (PBS ip.) the SNT detected a positive antibody titer.

Discussion

Serological techniques are successfully used for diagnosis of viral diseases in mammals, for instance, for the Vesicular Stomatitis Virus (VSV), also a rhabdovirus like VHSV, that cause vesicular disease of horses, cattle and pigs [25]. In fish, however, development and validation of serological methods for diagnosis of viral diseases is clearly less advanced than in mammals, although there would be a great demand in routine diagnostics. In the case of VHS, several serological methods have been described in the literature, but currently there exists no gold standard. In addition to this lack on the side of the diagnostic methodology, a factor that further complicates the evaluation and validation of serological methods for VHS is the lack of a reliable and reproducible infection model that would provide sera known to be positive for *anti*-VHSV- antibodies. Therefore, when initiating the present study, we were confronted with two tasks: first, to compare different methods of infecting fish with VHSV, and second to evaluate the performance of serological methods in detecting *anti*-VHSV antibodies in fish subjected to VHSV with the different infection methods.

Three different serological methods for detection of anti-VHSV antibodies were used in the present study: two ELISAs, an indirect one and an antigen capture ELISA, and a SNT which relies on a detection principle different to that of the ELISAs. Since we tested aliquots of the same individuals in all three assays, a direct comparison of the test results per individual fish was possible (s. Tabs.5-7). With this approach, we found mismatches between the results of the serological methods in classifying sero-positive and sero-negative fish. In comparing the results obtained by the ELISA techniques for the groups B11 (ip.), B12 (ip.+rect.), and B13 (rect.), the capture ELISA apparently detected nearly twice as many fish with positive sera than the indirect ELISA. Further, whereas the capture ELISA resulted in a clear ranking with respect to the number of the sero-positive fish from group B11 over group B12 to group B13, the indirect ELISA found less pronounced group differences, with the numbers of sero-positive fish being identical in the two groups B12 and B13 and an only slightly higher sero-prevalence for group B11 (s. Tab.8). Mismatches between the two ELISA techniques seemed to be unidirectional, because sera, which were tested positive with the indirect ELISA, were also positive in the capture ELISA (with one exception) whereas only 51% of the sera, found positive in the capture ELISA, were also positive in the indirect ELISA. With other words: the capture ELISA revealed a higher sero-prevalence than the indirect ELISA. This leads to the question, whether the capture ELISA provides false-positives or whether the indirect ELISA generates false-negatives?

To approach this question, we re-examined the criteria by which the two ELISAs discriminate sero-positive and sero-negative probes. Since the indirect ELISA showed a lower number of sero-positive fish than the capture ELISA, the question was whether our calculated threshold for positive samples in the indirect ELISA may be too conservative. When the threshold of the indirect ELISA (s. Materials and Methods), which in our hands was 0.095 OD, is arbitrarily lowered by 25 % to 0.072, only 2 out of 19 mismatches between the two ELISA protocols disappeared (Tab.8). With the threshold of 0.072, no sera of control fish (B9, B14, baseline) became not yet positive, but further reducing the threshold would increase the risk of false-positives. Overall, a 25 % reduction of the threshold did not substantially reduce the mismatches between the two ELISA protocols. The same happened when we reduced the sensitivity of the capture ELISA by elevating the threshold of this assay.

Table 8: Results of indirect ELISA (indirect) and capture ELISA (capture) after changing the thresholds for discrimination between sero-positive and sero-negative sample: capture ELISA: only values ≥640 titer as positives; indirect ELISA: all values over 0.072 absorbance as positives. Sera are correlated to Tabs.5+6. To simplify the demonstration, ELISA values were turned into yes-no-answers.

fish-no.	B9		B10		B11		B12		B13		B14	
	capture	indirect	capture	indirect	capture	indirect	capture	indirect	capture	Indirect	capture	indirect
1	0	0		1	1	1	0		0	0	0	0
2	0	0	0	1	0	0	0	0	1	1	0	0
3	0	0	1	1	1	0	1	1	0	0	0	0
4	0	0	1	1	1	1	0	0	0	0	0	0
5	0	0	1	1	0	0	0	0	1	1	0	0
6	0	0	1	1	0	0	1	1	0	0	0	0
7	0	0	0	0	1	1	0	0	1	0	0	0
8	0	0	1	0	1	0	1	0	0	0	0	0
9	0	0	1	1	0	0	1	0		0	1	0
10			1	0	0	0	1	0	0	0	0	0
11			1	1	1	1	0	0	0	0	0	0
12			0	1	1	1	0	0	1	1	0	0
13			1	1	0	0	1	0	0	0	0	0
14			1	1	0	0	1	0	0	0	0	0
15				1	1	0	0	0	0	0	0	0
16			1	1	1	1		1		1		
17			0	1	1	1				1		
18				1						0		
19				1						0		
20				0						0		
			11/15	16/20	10/17	7/17	7/15	3/16	4/15	5/20	1/15	
			73%	80%	59%	41%	47%	19%	27%	25%	7%	

1= positive; 0= negative

B9: infected with Y. ruckeri; B10: ip.-infected twice with VHSV; B11: ip.-infected with VHSV; B12: ip.+ rect.-infected with VHSV; B13: rect.-infected with VHSV; B14: ip.-injected with PBS

Again, the number of mismatches was reduced by two sera, i.e. the effect of hanging the threshold was only marginal (Tab.8). The only minimal increase in concordance between the two methods by altering the thresholds would suggest, that there are other reasons for unconformity than thresholds.

All serological tests did not detect any positive *anti*-VHSV antibody titers in the control groups B9 and the baseline group (day 0). With one exception in SNT and capture ELISA, also the PBS-infected group B14 was shown to be sero-negative. These findings indicate that the serological assays are specific.

As a further serological test, we used the SNT since this assay has a different detection principle than ELISA. While the latter method relies on antibody-antigen interaction, the SNT is measuring complement-dependent neutralization of virus by antibodies. The overall concordance between the three assays was 70 % hence in 30 % of the fish the three assays did not match. There was no tendency that the SNT results were more in accordance with one of the two ELISA methods, but it was more or less equidistant to both, the indirect an the capture ELISA: The number of mismatches of the SNT to the indirect ELISA was 23 % and to the capture ELISA 24 %. There are only few reports about direct comparisons between an indirect ELISA technique and a SNT, that all described differences in the percentages of detection of sero-positives [9-11,26]. The differences of percentages of sero-positives varied from 10 %, in fish challenged under experimental conditions [10], and 30 % in fish under field conditions [9]. One report found no correlations between the used ELISA and SNT methods at all [11]. Due to that, detection of less sero-positives with SNT than with ELISA techniques was expected at the beginning of the experiment. Thus, in contrast to previous reports, we mainly compared two ELISAs and used the SNT as control test, but there were no correlations found between two tests in the mismatching sera. Therefore, the SNT does not help in answering the question on what samples are false positive or false negative.

The percentage of mismatches between ELISAs and SNT may vary for the different infection methods [9,10]. From our results the number of mismatches seemed to be lower in group B13 (rect.) than in the other groups. However, the overall n-numbers were too small to come to firm conclusions on whether this is a true treatment effect or not. A clear treatment effect was indicated for the booster group B10, however this effect was expressed more in an elevation of the antibody titer rather than in an increase of the number of sero-positive fish.

Another parameter, that could possibly give more information about the serological status of the challenged groups thereby helping to answer the question which ELISA is more accurate, is the prevalence of virus-positive fish per group (Tab.9). Theoretically, one might expect that viro-prevalence correlates with sero-prevalence, but this expectation is not unequivocally supported by our data. Summing up the results of the virological assays (RT-PCR and virus re-isolation), there was a clear ranking between a very low virus-prevalence in group B13 (rect.) and much higher virus-prevalence in groups B11 (ip.) and B12 (ip. + rect.), the latter two groups showing no clear differences. Successful detection of VHSV after challenging rainbow trout with VHSV by ip.-injection was described before [7,17], but rarely viro-prevalence was checked as an indication for sero-prevalence [9]. The challenge of fish with VHSV by only rectal application resulting in sero-positive fish was not described before, only in combination with ip.-injection [8]. In terms of sero-prevalence, there is more a grade change between the treatments: The serological assays yielded a ranking of sero-prevalence of B11 > B12 > B13, what is in contrast to the ranking according to viro-prevalence which is B11 ≅ B12 >> B13. Remarkably, the viro-prevalence in group B13 was about one order of magnitude lower than the sero-prevalence - a finding that is clearly in contrast to the other treatments. In summing up, the correlation of prevalence of virus and prevalence of *anti*-VHSV-antibodies seemed to be limited, at its best there is a tendency that higher viro-prevalence associates with elevated sero-prevalence.

Table 9: Overview of positive organ samples, tested to VHSV with re-isolation method (re-isol.) and PCR versus positive serological results with capture ELISA (capture), indirect ELISA (indirect) and SNT in percentages on group levels.

	B10	B11	B12	B13
re-isol.	20	50	40	3
PCR	40	60	63	3
capture	80	71	53	33
indirect	65	38	20	20
SNT	67	71	33	20

B10: ip.-challenged boosted
B11: ip.-challenged once
B12: ip.+ rect.-challenged
B13: rect. -challenged

This study aimed to compare various techniques and infection methods but was not designed to examine the causes for the mismatches between the treatments. Thus, we can only speculate on possible explanations. One explanation could be related to methodological problems. In the two ELISAs, identical sera were tested using the same virus and the same antibody against *anti*-VHSV antibodies (Mab 4C10). This suggests that the mismatches are not due to differences in the key antibody-antigen reaction, e.g., because of different specificities or affinities of the primary antibodies, but the cause for the between-method variation should be sought in methodological aspects of the two protocols. The indirect ELISA may be more sensitive than the capture ELISA to variations in the quality of the purified virus. During virus purification, the trans-membrane glycoprotein (G protein) as a major antigenic site of the VHS-virus [8,18,26,27,30] can get lost. This loss of G protein may strongly limits the detection-capacity of the indirect ELISA, because the major part of *anti*-VHSV antibodies are binding with this antigen. This problem is avoided in the capture ELISA by fixing the virus with polyclonal antibodies on the plate. Another possible flaw in the indirect ELISA might be the direct virus coating on microplates that can vary with the microplate binding capacities, which again can vary from lot to lot. In the capture ELISA protocol, a potential methodological weakness was the high non-specific binding of fish sera, what increases the background absorbance, and may lead to false positives. In the capture ELISA, for detection of the antigenic determinate, a mixture of two monoclonal *anti*-trout antibodies (Mab D_2, Mab 4C10) was used. Due to that, detection signal may be enhanced, what could lead to the higher number of sero-positives found with the capture ELISA. However, in comparative measurements using the mixture and single monoclonal antibodies, an unequivocal influence of the mixture could not be observed (NJ Olesen, pers. communication). This leads us to the other possible factor causing mismatches, that is the biology of antibodies and their interactions with other serum proteins. The explanation of the underlying reasons for the assay mismatches is complicated by the insufficient knowledge of the fish immune response, in particular the adaptive immune system, to virus infections [13,16,26-31]. Without knowing sufficiently well the elements and mechanisms involved in the antiviral response of the fish, it is difficult to understand why differences in assay protocols could result in different classifications of positive and negative sera. Published data revealed that the susceptibility to pathogenic agents and the subsequent induction of the immune response in fish showed a highly individual variation [9,10,14]. This became again evident from the data of this study, particularly from the results of virus re-isolation, respectively virus RNA isolation with RT-PCR, in group B10 and B11. Due to this high inter-individual variation sampling size for serological studies must be large enough.

Conclusion

Given the fact that neither established infection models nor serological techniques for diagnosis of VHS disease in salmonids are available, the present study aimed for a comparative evaluation of methods to infect rainbow trout with VHSV and to detect anti-VHSV antibodies in trout serum. The key findings are:

- the prevalence of infected fish, as diagnosed by direct virus detection (virus re-isolation, RT-PCR) varied with the infection method: Intra-peritoneal injections, either single or as booster injection or in combination with rectal infection, gave higher prevalence than rectal infection. However, with none of the methods, a 100 % prevalence was achieved. This inability to generate a defined prevalence complicates the interpretation of serological assays.
- even if we would be able to generate a defined VHS prevalence by any of the infection methods, the results form this study indicate that there is no straightforward relation between the percentage of fish tested positive in the direct virus detection (virus re-isolation, RT-PCR) and the percentage of sero-positive fish. The high percentages of viro-prevalence were all about the same in the intra-peritoneal injected and the intra-peritoneal plus rectal appliquéd groups (B11,B12), but the only rectal appliquéd group was clearly underestimated by direct virus detection methods in comparison to the nearly ten times higher percentages of sero-prevalence.
- the results of the three serological methods used in this study (capture ELISA, indirect ELISA, SNT) agreed for 70 % of the analyzed sera, but yielded differing results for 30 % of the sera. The capture ELISA and the SNT tended to give more positive sera than the indirect ELISA, however, at the current state of knowledge we have no criteria to decide which results are false positives or false negatives.

Taken together, these findings suggest that the use serological approaches for monitoring and supervising the VHS status of fish stocks is too premature. Further, our results point to an insufficient understanding on those factors in the virus-host interaction that decide on a successful infection of the fish.

References

[1] Jensen MH. 1963. Preparation of fish tissue cultures for virus research. Bull off int Epiz 59: 131-134.

[2] Zwillenberg LO, Jensen MH, Zwillenberg HHL. 1965. Electron microscopy of the virus of viral haemorrhagic septicaemia of rainbow trout (Egtved virus). Arch ges Virusforsch 17: 1-19.

[3] Van Regenmortel MHV, Fauquet CM, Bishop DHL, Carstens EB and 7 others. 2000. Virus taxonomy: classification and nomenclature of viruses-seventh report of international comitee on taxonomy of viruses. Academic Press, San Diego, CA.

[4] Office International des Epizooties. 2006. Diagnostic Manual of Aquatic Animal Diseases. Office International des Epizooties capt. 2.1.5.

[5] Anonymous. Commission Decision 2001/183/EC, Annex, Part III and IV, 2001.

[6] Anonymus. 1995. Swiss Federal Animal Health Ordinance: SR 916.401 chapt. 5, Art. 1-4.

[7] López-Vàzquez C, Dopazo CP, Olveira JG, Barja JL, Bandín I. 2005. Development of a rapid, sensitive and non-lethal diagnostic assay for the detection of viral haemorrhagic septicaemia virus. J Virol Methods 133: 167-174.

[8] Utke K, Bergmann S, Lorenzen N, Köllner B, Ototake M, Fischer U. 2007. Cell-mediated cytotoxicity in raibow trout, *Oncorhynchus mykiss*, infected with viral haemorrhagic septicaemia virus. Fish Shellfish Immunol 22: 182-196.

[9] Fregeneda-Grandes JM, Olesen NJ. Detection of rainbow trout antibodies against viral haemorrhagic septicaemia virus (VHSV) by neutralisation test is highly dependent on the virus isolate used. Dis Aquat Org 74: 151-158.

[10] Olesen NJ, Lorenzen N, Jørgensen PEV. 1991. Detection of rainbow trout antibody to Egtved virus by enzyme-linked immunosorbent assay (ELISA), immunofluorescence (IF), and plaque neutralization test (50%PNT). Dis Aquat Org 10:31-38.

[11] Cossarini-Dunier M. 1985. Indirect Enzyme-Linked Immunosorbent Assey (ELISA) to titrate rainbow trout serum antibodies against two pathogens: *Yersinia ruckeri* and Egtved Virus. Aquaculture 49: 197-208.

[12] Knüsel R, Segner H, Wahli T. 2003. A survey of viral diseases in farmed and feral salmonids in Switzerland. J Fish Diseas 26: 167-182.

[13] Fernandez-Alonso M, Alvarez F, Estepa A, Coll JM. 1999. G disulphide bond native conformation is required to elicit trout neutralizing antibodies against VHSV. J Fish Diseas 22:219-222.

[14] Hattenberger-Baudouy AM, Danton M, Merle G, de Kinkelin P. 1995. Serum neutralization test for epidemiological studies of salmonid rhabdoviroses in France. Vet Res 26: 512-520.

[15] Enzmann PJ, Konrad M. 1993. Longevity of antibodies in brown trout and rainbow trout following experimental infection with VHS-Virus. Bull Eur Ass Fish Pathol 13(6): 193.

[16] Enzmann PJ, Bruchhof B. 1989. Comparative studies on viral hemorrhagic septicemia viruses and infectious hematopoietic necrosis virus. An attempt to demonstrate an immunological relationship. In: Lillelung K, Rosenthal H, editors. Fish health protection strategies. Bonn, Germany: Bundesministerium für Forschung und Technologie. p.107-120.

[17] Ortega C, Milani A, Muzquiz JL, Alonso JL, Simon MC, Garcia J, Girones O, Graselli A. 1992. Comparative study of the fluorescent antibody technique and cell culture isolation in the diagnostic of haemorrhagic septicaemia. Bull Eur Ass Fish Pathol 12(6): 191-192.

[18] Boudinot P, Blanco M, de Kinkelin P, Benmansour A. 1998. Combined DNA Immunization with the Glycoprotein Gene of Viral Hemorrhagic Septicemia Virus and Infectious Hematopoietic Necrosis Virus Induces Double-Specific Protective Immunity and Nonspecific Response in Rainbow Trout. Virology 249: 297-306.

[19] Olesen NJ, Jørgensen PEV. 1991. Rapid detection of viral haemorrhagic septicaemia virus in fish by ELISA. J Appl Ichthyol 7: 183-186.

[20] Bergmann SM, Olesen NJ, Frank Skall H, Einer-Jensen K, Fichtner D. Dis Aquat Org. submitted.

[21] Knüsel R, Bergmann S, Einer-Jensen K, Casey J, Segner H, Wahli T. 2007. Virus isolation versus RT-PCR: Which method is more successful in detecting VHSV and IHNV in fish tissue sampled under field conditions?. J Fish Diseas 30: 559-568.

[22] Thuvander A, Fossum C, Lorenzen N. 1990. Monoclonal antibodies to samlonid immunglobulin: characterization and applicability in immunoasseys. Dev Comp Immunol 14: 415-423.

[23] Hintze J. 2006. NCSS, PASS, and GESS. NCSS. Kaysville, Utah. WWW.NCSS.COM.

[24] Roberts RJ. 1989. Fish Pathology. Baillière Tindall, London, England.

[25] Office International des Epizooties. 2004. Manual of Diagnostic Tests and Vaccines for Terrestrial Animals. Office International des Epizooties capt. 2.1.2.

[26] Lorenzen N, Lapatra SE. 1999. Immunity to rhabdoviruses in rainbow trout: the antibody response. Fish Shellfish Immunol 9: 345-360.

[27] Lorenzen N, Olesen NJ, Jørgensen PEV. 1993. Antibody response to VHS virus proteins in rainbow trout. Fish Shellfish Immunol 3: 461-473.

[28] Bird S, Zou J, Secombes C. 2006. Advances in fish cytokine biology give clues to the evolution of a complex network. Curr Phar Des 12: 3051-3069.

[29] Bernstein RM, Schluter SF, Marchalonis JJ. 1998. Immunity. In: Evans DH, editor. The Physiology of Fish. CRC Press LLC, USA. p. 215-245.

[30] Bachmann MF, Zinkernagel RM. 1996. The influence of virus structure on antibody responses and virus serotype formation. Immunol Today 17:553-558.

[31] Köllner B, Wasserrab B, Kotterba G, Fischer U. 2002. Evaluation of immune functions of rainbow trout (*Oncorhynchus mykiss*) – how can environmental influences be detected?. Toxicol Lett 131: 83-95.

Dank

Zum Schluss komme ich zum wohl schönsten, weil letzten, aber auch schwierigsten Teil meiner Arbeit. Schwierig deshalb, weil es, wenn ich alle Menschen hier nennen dürfte, denen ich es zu verdanken habe, dass ich heute hier angelangt bin, der längste Teil von allen werden würde. Daher entschuldige ich mich schon jetzt, bei allen nicht persönlich genannten Freunden, Verwandten und Kollegen, die hoffentlich wissen, dass ihre Rollen zum Entstehen dieser Arbeit vielleicht nicht ganz so wichtig waren, wohl aber für mein ganzes Leben.

Allen voran verdanke ich es Prof. Helmut Segner, dessen Ruf als gefürchteter Korrekturleser zwar auch mich ereilte ☺, dass diese Arbeit hier und heute und in dieser Qualität fertig gestellt wurde. Denn wenn man plötzlich mit dem Rücken an der Wand steht, kann man sich darauf verlassen, dass er noch hinter einem steht.

Ebenso auch Dr. Thomas Wahli, dessen kompetente und fürsorgliche Betreuung seiner Doktoranden immer weit über das Fachliche hinaus geht.

Allen Mitarbeitern des FLI in Riems, die mich so freundlich aufgenommen und mich mit Wissen und Taten so kräftig unterstützt haben, allen voran Dr. Sven Bergmann, Frau Irina Werner, Dr. Dieter Fichtner, Dr. Bernd Köllner, Dr. Uwe Fichtner, Dr. Heike Schütze und meine Dani/Daniela Schrudde! ☺

Mange tak to all my most favourite Danes at the DTU, Niels Jørgen Olesen, Mette Eliassen, Nicole Nicolajsen, Helle Frank Skall, Niels Lorenzen and all the other amazing Århusers, who helped me so much and made me never forget my great times spending there!

Encore un grand merci à Dr. Jeannette Castric, qui par son aide rapide et opportune, a beaucoup contribué à mon étude.

Frau Professor Dr. Maja Suter für die freundliche Aufnahme im Institut der Tierpathologie.

Grosser Dank gebührt auch unseren Laborantinnen: Elisabeth Oldenberg, für ihre bewundernswerte Akkuratheit und ganz herzlich Barbara Müller, dem Wunder an universell einsetzbarer Effizienz. Der Fischebluten-Weltrekord ist unser!

Und natürlich meinen lieben Mitdoktoranden und Mitstreitern im tägliche Kampf gegen das Böse: Kathrin Bettge, Heike Schmidt-Posthaus, Sibylle Kipfer, Michael/Mix/BöserMichi!/Michel Wenger, Manu Weber, Daniel Bernet, Ayako Nakayama, Dmitri Pugovkin, Catharina Lany, Anja Möller, und Richi Burki, der unseren Schwarm leider, leider verlassen hat, aber immer einer der unseren bleibt.

Nicht unerwähnt sollen auch die Menschen sein, die mir ganz uneigennützig, aus reiner Kollegialität und Freundlichkeit geholfen haben, wie Joachim Müller und all die anderen lieben Kollegen aus der Parasitologie, sowie Dr. Reto Zanoni und den lieben Laborantinnen der Virologie, und auch Dr. Joachim Enzmann.

Mein tiefster Dank gilt auch meinen Eltern, Gisela und Werner Klenk, ohne die ich niemals hier angekommen wäre, sowie Matthias und Alexander, die ihren Job als grosse Brüder wohl auch ganz gut gemacht haben, in der Schulung aufs Leben. ☺

Und zuletzt möchte ich noch bei ein paar Freunde bedanken, die mir schon seit so langer, und auch erst kürzer Zeit, zur Seite gestanden haben: Bettina ehemals Bittner, Bianca-Marie Weimar, die Teams der VoKli 2003/04/05 - Wiege meines eigentlichen Lebens als Tierarzt - Danke für die Hammer Zeiten!, Familie Drees, Kess/Kerstin Schlüter, Peter Giger, meinem persönlichen (Formatierungs-)Helden, und noch einmal dir, Kathi, denn wir sind das vereinte deutsche Volk und wir schaffen das! ☺

Und meinem liebsten Schatz Marcel Rindlisbacher!

Methodensammlung

Herstellung von Penicillin G-Portionen 1Mio IE

Begriffe, Definitionen und Abkürzungen:
AB   Antibiotika
IE   Internationale Einheiten

4. Notwendiges Material

Lösungen/Substanzen	Penicillin G-Portion à 10^6 IE	-15 bis -35°C, T010
	Amphotericin B steril	-15 bis -35°C
	Streptophenat steril	2-8°C
	Aqua bidest steril	
Geräte/Material	sterile Spritze 5ml u. Kanüle	
	sterile 100ml Glasflaschen	
	Flammatic	
	steriler Erlenmeyer 1l	
	Tiefkühlschrank –15 bis -35°C	
	Kühlschränke 2-8°C	
	15ml-Polypropylen-Röhrchen mit Deckel	

5. Methodenbeschrieb

5.1 In Flowbench 1g Streptophenat in sterilem Aqua bidest. vorlösen: Mit steriler Spritze ca. 3ml steriles Aqua bidest. in Fläschchen mit lyophilisiertem Streptophenat geben, mischen und über Flammatic leicht erwärmen, bis sich das Streptophenat löst. Diese Lösung mit Spritze herausziehen und in sterilen Erlenmeyer geben.
5.2 Streptophenat-Fläschchen mit ca. 3ml sterilem Aqua bidest nachspülen und dies ebenfalls in den Erlenmeyer geben.
5.3 10ml steriles Amphotericin B in Erlenmeyer pipettieren
5.4 Penicillin G-Portion à 10^6 IE in Erlenmeyer geben
5.5 Auffüllen mit sterilem Aqua bidest. ad. 1l
5.6 Gut mischen und in 100ml-Portionen in sterile Glasflaschen abfüllen und beschriften: AB, Chargen-Nr., Herstellungsdatum, Verfalldatum und Visum
5.7 Flaschen nicht fest verschliessen, mit abgeflammter Alufolie Schraubverschluss abdecken und sofort in Tiefkühlschrank bei einer Temperatur –15 bis –35°C in Schrägstellung einfrieren (Haltbarkeit: 2 Jahre)
5.8 AB-Lösung in Chargen-Protokoll (f-m-v001-01) eintragen
5.9 Sobald die AB-Lösung gefroren ist, Flaschen ganz verschliessen
5.10 Nach Bedarf aus einer 100ml-Portion 4.5ml Portionen in Polypropylen-Röhrchen mit Deckel abfüllen. Diese bei 2-8°C aufbewahren (Haltbarkeit 1 Jahr).

Komplement aus Fischserum für SNT (Serumneutralisationstest)

Begriffe, Definitionen und Abkürzungen:
SPNT: Serum-Plaques-Neutralisationstest
Cryo Tubes: Sterile Spezial-Röhrchen mit Schraubverschluss
Komplement: Thermolabiler Serumfaktor. der sowohl bei unspezifischen Abwehrvorgängen als auch bei Immunreaktionen eine grosse Rolle spielt.

4. Notwendiges Material

Prüfungsmaterial	Fische
Geräte/Material	Kühlzentrifuge
	Zentrifugenröhrchen
	Spritzen und Kanülen
	Sterilfilter Acrodisc 0,45µm
	Kühlschrank
	Cryo Tubes
	Eisbad
	Kühlzentrifuge

5. Methodenbeschrieb

5.1 Möglichst grosse Fische (Mutterfische) mit Genickschlag töten.
5.2 Fisch auf Rücken legen und Kanüle hinter der Afterflosse schräg Richtung Kopf gegen Wirbelsäule einstechen, bis Knochen spürbar ist; dann die Kanüle ein wenig zurückziehen und das Blut aspirieren. Solange Blut nehmen, wie dieses gut fliesst.
5.3 Blut in Zentrifugenröhrchen einfüllen.
5.4 Das Blut 1 Stunden bei Raumtemperatur, anschliessend über Nacht bei 2-8°C im Kühlschrank gerinnen lassen.
5.5 Nach Gerinnung den Blutkuchen mit einem Spatel vom Rand lösen.
5.6 Blut in Kühlzentrifuge D002 bei Temperatureinstellung 4°C, und Toureneinstellung 3'500 während 10 Minuten zentrifugieren.
5.7 Das von diesem Zeitpunkt an benötigte Material, soll im Eisbad vorgekühlt werden. Das gesamte Serum eines Fisches wird mittels Acrodisc-Sterilfilter (0,45µm) sterilfiltriert. Seren verschiedener Fische sollen nicht gemischt werden (erhöhte Koagulationsbereitschaft der Komplemente)
5.8 In Portionen à 1ml in Cryo-Tubes bei tiefer als –65°C lagern.

6. Anmerkungen

Bei der Serumgewinnung ist darauf zu achten, dass das Blut nicht länger als 60 Minuten bei Zimmertemperatur gehalten wird, da Komplement sehr wärmeempfindlich ist.

Titration und Auszählung von Fischviren nach der Kärber Methode

Begriffe, Definitionen und Abkürzungen:

DVL	Danish Veterinary Laboratory
BF	Bluegill Fry Zell-Linien
EPC	Epithelioma Papulosa Carpio Zell-Linien
VHS	Virale Hämorrhagische Septikämie
IHN	Infektiöse Hämatopoetische Nekrose
IPN	Infektiöse Pankreas-Nekrose
SVC	Frühlings-Virämie der Karpfen
EU	Europäische Union

3. Notwendiges Material

Prüfmaterial	Fischviren
Zellen	EPC auf Mikrotiter-Platte mindestens 8, höchstens 48 Std. nach Einsaat für IHN-, VHS, IPN u. SVC
	BF auf Mikrotiter-Platte mindestens 8, höchstens 48 Std. nach Einsaat für VHS, IPN u. SVC
Lösungen Geräte/Material	MEM Wachstumsmedium mit Trispuffer
	Mikrotiterplatten
	Multichannel-Kolbenhubpipette
	Flow-Bench
	Inkubator 13-17°C
	Tiefkühlschrank tiefer als -65°C

4. Methodenbeschrieb

Redissolve the lyophilizied material carefully in 2.00 ml cell culture medium (Eagle MEM) supplemented with 10% fetal calf serum (FCS) and TRIS buffer, filter through 0.45 μm membrane filter and transfer the solution to sterile tubes.
For dilution use 96-well microtiter plates with round bottoms (e.g. Micro well Plates, Life Technologies).
  1. Transfer 180 μl cell culture medium with 10% FCS and TRIS buffer to the 7 bottom wells in each collum (2 x 7 wells per virus)
  2. Transfer 200 μl undiluted virus to the first well in 2 collums
  3. With a multichannel pipette adjusted to 20 μl (if available) dip tips in a row A (undiluted virus), mix 20 times and transfer 20 μl to the surface of the medium in the wells of row B (without dipping the tip into the medium). Put on new tips, dip into wells in row B, mix 20 times and transfer 20 μl to the surface of the medium in the ells of row C, and so on

For each ampoule, use a 96-well cell culture plate with 24 h old BF-2 cells ($^1/_2$ plate) and EPC cells ($^1/_2$ plate). A seeding density of 50.000 to 100.000 cells per well, in our laboratory results in approximately 80% confluence after 24 h in incubation at 20°C, but this may vary to others. Use normal cell culture medium (s.a. plus antibiotics), 150 µl per well.
Inoculate 25 µl/well of each virus dilution into 6 replicate wells for each cell line, using a multichannel pipette. Inoculate 3 replicates from each column in the dilution plate onto each cell line.
Incubate at 15°C until final reading 7 days after inoculation, where wells with CPE are registered.

Virus titration using Kärber method:

the titre of the virus is : R^T
it is expressed in $TCID_{50}$ (dose giving 50 % effect) /unit of volume

$$T = d + \left[\frac{r}{N} \times \left(n + \frac{N}{2} \right) \right]$$

with

    d :   negative log of the lowest dilution giving a 100 % positive response
    r :   log R (R = dilution interval)
    N :   number of wells/dilution
    n :   number of wells giving a ⊕ response (the dilutions where all wells give 0 % or 100 % response are not taking into account)

Exemple of calculation of viral titre by Kärber method:

(Dilutions from 10 to 10 ; 4 wells/dilution)

Dilution	Number of positive wells	Number of negative wells
10-3	4	0
10-4	4	0
10-5	4	0
10-6	4	0
10-7	3	1
10-8	2	2
10-9	0	4

$$T = d + \left[\frac{r}{N} \times \left(n + \frac{N}{2} \right) \right]$$

$$T = d + \left[\frac{1}{4} \times \left(n + \frac{4}{2} \right) \right]$$

$$T = d + \left(\frac{n+2}{4} \right)$$

$d = 6$
$r = 1$
$N = 4$
$n = 5$

$$T = 6 + \left[\frac{1}{4} \times \left(5 + \frac{4}{2} \right) \right] \qquad T = 6 + \frac{7}{4} = 7,75$$

viral titre= $10^{7,75}$ $TCID_{50}$/unit of tested volume

If tested volume is 100 µl/well (24 well plate) : Viral titre = $10^{8.75}$ $TCID_{50}$/ml

If tested volume is 25 µl /well (96 well plate) : Viral titre = $4.10^{8.75}$ $TCID_{50}$/ml

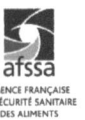

End point seroneutralisation test (SNT) for detection of anti-VHSV antibodies

I Titration of the reference VHSV used in the SNT

The reference VHSV strain used in the SNT is the isolate 07/71 from diseased rainbow trout. The virus stock, grown in EPC cells and used for SNT is aliquoted by 0.5 ml and kept at −80°C. An aliquot of the virus is thawed for virus titration in a 96 well-plate containing EPC cells, using an end point dilution technique.
Serial tenfold dilutions of the virus (from 10^{-1} to 10^{-8}) are prepared by transferring 20µl of virus in tubes containing 180 µl of cell culture medium. Then 25 µl of each dilution are inoculated in the corresponding wells of a 96 well-microplate containing 24 to 48 hours old EPC cells (at least 4 wells per dilution). The plates are incubated at 14°C +/- 1°C during 4 to 6 days. Then the cells are fixed and stained using cristal violet solution in ethanol and the infectious titre evaluated using Kärber formula in $TCID_{50}$/ml *(see annex 1)*.

II Seroneutralisation test

1- Preparation of the cells in flat bottom 96-wells microplates

EPC cells are prepared 24 to 48 hours before inoculation.
> Prepare 15 ml of cell suspension containing 20.10^6 cells for each plate and distribute 150 µl of cell suspension in each well of a 96 well-plate.
> Incubate the cells at 29°C +/- 2°C for 24 to 48 hours.

Number of plates to prepare : twin plates are prepared for each serie of sera or plasma and for the controls.

> If the objective of the test is to know the number of seropositive fish among a population, 2 plates are used for 20 sera diluted from 1/40 to 1/320.
> If the objective is to evaluate the neutralising titre, then dilutions from 1/40 to 1/5120 (or more) are used and the number of plates is 2 for 10 sera.

2- Sera or plasma dilutions in round bottom 96-wells microplates ; plan twin plates for each serie of sera

The sera to be tested must have been de-complemented by heat treatment at 45°C for 30 min.

> Sera or plasma are diluted in a twofold dilution series across the plates using cell culture medium.

The first dilution 1/20 (20µl serum + 380µl medium) can be done in tubes on a racket having the same size as a microplate, so that a multichannel pipette can be used to distribute the 1/20 dilution from the tubes to the first row of a microplate. The tubes containing the dilutions 1/10 and 1/20 can then be maintained at 5°C +/- 3°C until the end of the analysis.

In case of any problem during the analysis, those tubes can be used to perform the test again.

> Dispense 30 µl of cell culture medium in all the wells of each plate.

- Dispense 30 µl of each serum diluted 1/20 in the corresponding wells of the first line of the twin plates and mix 10 times by sucking in and out using the multichannel pipette = dilution 1/40
- Then, without changing the tips, transfer 30 µl of sera from the first line to the second one, mix 10 times... = dilution 1/80.
- Continue until dilution 1/320 (for a routine control) or higher if the neutralising titre of the serum must be evaluated.
- Discard 30 µl from the last row, after dilution.

3 – Control plates (in twin plates)

The following controls must be prepared :
- EPC cells control : 60µl cell culture medium /well
- EPC cells + complement : 30µl cell culture medium + 30µl of the medium used for virus dilution /well
- Reference VHSV 07/71 : 30µl cell culture medium /well
- Negative anti-VHSV serum : 30µl of diluted serum (dilution 1/40 to 1/320) /well
- Standard anti-VHSV serum of known titre: 30µl of diluted serum (dilution 1/80 to 1/10240 or more) /well

4 – virus preparation and addition in the plates

For each plate, prepare 3ml of viral suspension of VHSV (07/71) containing about 6.10^4 $TCID_{50}$.
The virus is diluted in cell culture medium containing complement at a final dilution of 1/20.

This virus suspension is kept in ice during the assay.

- Add 30µl of viral suspension (about 600 $TCID_{50}$) in each well of the plates containing the sera to test and in a part of the control plates (reference virus, negative and positive sera dilutions),

For the sera to be tested, begin by the highest dilution so that there is no need to change tips between each row.
For the control plates, begin by the positive serum then change tips for the negative serum, then change tips for the control virus
- Shake gently the plates for about 5 mn

5 – incubation and transfer

- Incubate the plates at 5°C +/- 3°C for 16 to 24 h
- Transfer 50µl from the wells of the SN plates to the corresponding wells of the plates containing EPC cells.
- Begin by the highest dilution of sera until the lowest without changing tips
- Incubate the plates at 14°C +/- 1°C during 3 to 4 days

6 – fixation and staining

After 3 days incubation, observe a control plate using an inverted microscope:
- The cell control must be intact

- The cell sheet in the virus control must be destroyed at 75 to 90% compared to the cell control

- The standard positive control serum has a neutralising titre close to the value expected.

If those conditions are met, fix and stain one of the control plates by discarding the medium and using about 50 µl of crystal violet solution (1.3 g crystal violet powder dissolved in 100 ml ethanol + 400 ml water) for at least 1 hour. Then discard the colorant, rinse the plates with tap water until the color of the water is pale purple and let them drying at room temperature.

Depending on the degree of sheet destruction in the virus control, one additionnal day incubation may be necessary.

7 – reading and interpretation

➢ conditions to be fulfilled in order to get interpretable results :

- Cell control : correct sheet with and without complement
- Control virus : 75 to 90% destruction of the cell sheet
- Control negative serum : same destruction as in the control virus
- Standard positive serum : neutralising titre as expected (+/- one dilution)

Sera to test :
        Neutralising titre is the inverse of the initial serum dilution giving 50% neutralisation of the reference VHSV compared to the control virus.

Threshold sensitivity : 1/80

VHSV-Konzentrierung

1) Anzuchtmedium mit Zellen und Virus 3x auftauen und anschliessend wieder einfrieren. Mindestens 1l Anzuchtmedium für eine Virusaufreinigung verwenden. Alle Schritte der Viruskonzentrierung gekühlt auf Eis durchführen.

2) Aus Anzuchtmedium mit 5 000U über 15min bei 4°C den Zelldetritus entfernen. Zentrifuge: Centrikon T-124; Rotor: 6.9; 6x 500ml Flaschen (Virologie)

   Riems: mit 3000U/min über 10min

   Überstand aufbewahren! Zelldetritus in jeweils 1ml TNE-Puffer auflösen, und in Tubes umfüllen (auch poolbar). Anschliessend Tubes 2x für 30sec. in Ultraschallbad (Eisbad) tauchen um restliche Viren von Zellwand zu lösen. Überstand erneut in kleiner Zentrifuge trennen (Laborzentrifuge; 5 000U,15 min, 4°C) und zu anderem Überstand dazugeben.

3) Pelletierung des Überstands mit 20 000U über 1h45min bei 4°C.
   Zentrifuge: Centrikon T-2070; Rotor: TFA20.250; 6x 250ml Flaschen, füllen bis unter Flaschenhals (Virologie)

   Riems: im TFT 4595: 97 000g über 1h (26000U/min) oder TST 2838: 28 000U/min über 90min

   Überstand nach Zentrifugation verwerfen.

4) Pellet in TNE-Puffer (**pH 8,6**) aufnehmen.   TNE-Puffer: 0,02M Tries
   0,1M NaCl
   0,005M EDTA

   So viel TNE-Puffer verwenden, dass insgesamt 8 ml Pellet-Pufferlösung bleibt. Über Nacht auf Eis bei 4°C auflösen lassen.

5) Saccharosegradient 20%, 40%, 50% und 60% (schwerste zuunterst), am besten vorher fertig gestellt und in -80°C bis Gebrauch gelagert. Zum Gebrauch Saccharosegradient aufgetaut zuoberst mit Puffer-Pelletlösung bis ca. 3mm unter Röhrchenrand füllen. Dann mit 24 000U über 3h30min bei 10°C zentrifugieren.
   Zentrifuge: Centrikon T-2070; Rotor: AH629; 6x 38ml Röhrchen (Virologie)

   Riems: im TST 2838: 97 000g über 3h (26 000U/min)

6) Banden über Eierlampe (Virologie) aus Saccharose mit Pipette entnehmen. Obersten zwei 2-3 Banden (wichtigsten) zusammen in 50ml-Röhrchen aufnehmen.
   Zur Trennung aus der Saccharose bei 35 000U über 1h bei 4°C zentrifugieren. Röhrchen bis ca. 3mm untern Rand füllen, gegebenenfalls mit TNE-Puffer strecken.
   Zetrifuge: Centrikon T-2070; Rotor: AH641; 6x 13ml Röhrchen (Virologie)

   Riems: erneut Pelettieren im TST2838: 28 000U/min über 75min

   Überstand verwerfen.

7) Pellets in jeweils in 0,3ml TNE-Puffer aufnehmen und über Nacht auf Eis in Kühlschrank lösen lassen.

   Riems: (in 0,2-0,5mlTNE-Puffer)

   Am nächsten Tag mit Pipette vorsichtig lösen und Proteinbestimmung (NanoDrop) durchführen. Auf 3(-7) mg/ml Protein einstellen und bei -80°C bis Gebrauch lagern.

Indirekter ELISA nach Bergmann und Fichtner, FLI, Greifswald (Deutschland)

1) Ag-Absorption: 3µg/ml Virus in Absorptionspuffer (Carbonatpuffer pH: 8,6)
   (1:300 bzw. 33µl/10ml von Riemser Isolat)
   je 100µl pro Well über Nacht in 4°C
   Ausklopfen, nicht waschen!!

   Aufbewahrung: 5°C/feucht bis 1Jahr; -20°C über 1Jahr

   Schema: nur Absorptionsuffer - bleiben leer

A	1	2	3	4	5	6	7	8	9	10	11	12
B												
C												
D												
E												
F												
G												
H												

2) Blocken: Aqua dest. mit 1% Eialbumin oder Roti-Block (1:10 Verd.)
   je 200µl pro Well für 1h Zimmertemp. - danach waschen (2x kurz,1x lang (3 min) Einwirkzeit des Waschpuffers(WP)) und ausklopfen

   Schema: ganze Platte

A	1	2	3	4	5	6	7	8	9	10	11	12
B												
C												
D												
E												
F												
G												
H												

3) Serumtitration: Waschpuffer: je 100µl in Reihen B-H, Becher A1 und A12
Serumlösung: in Reihe B2-11 nochmal 200µl WP ergänzen, dann in Reihen B2-11 Serum 1:300 mit Waschpuffer (je 3µl Serum auf 300µl WP) mischen
aus Reihe B2-11 100µl in Reihe A2-11
und Reihe C2-11, von Reihe C jeweils 100µl in die darunter pipettieren
für 1h bei Zimmertemp. - danach waschen(s.o.) und ausklopfen

Schema:

A	1	2	3	4	5	6	7	8	9	10	11	12
B												
C												
D												
E												
F												
G												
H												

4) 2. Ak (anti-trout) den Mak 4C10 (Mouse) mit 1:200 in WP verdünnen
je 100µl pro Well für 1h bei Zimmertemp. - danach waschen

Schema: ganze Platte

A	1	2	3	4	5	6	7	8	9	10	11	12
B												
C												
D												
E												
F												
G												
H												

5) Konjugat (3.Ak)   einen anti-Mouse Phosphatase-gelabelten Ak mit WP
   Auf 1:10 000 (Pierce) oder 1:25 000 (Sigma) verdünnen
   je 100µl pro Well für 1h bei Zimmertemp. - danach waschen

   Schema: Zeile 1 nur **Waschpuffer**

	1	2	3	4	5	6	7	8	9	10	11	12
A												
B												
C												
D												
E												
F												
G												
H												

6) Substrat: 1 OPD-Tablette auf 10ml Phosphat-Citrat-Gemisch
   (Phosphat: 5.2ml und Citrat: 4.8ml)
   mit 10µl H_2O_2 (30%) aktivieren und je 100µl pro Well

   Schema: ganze Platte mit Substrat

	1	2	3	4	5	6	7	8	9	10	11	12
A												
B												
C												
D												
E												
F												
G												
H												

7) Stoppen: 50µl Schwefelsäure (4N) pro Well

Materialien für den indirekten ELISA

96-Platten von Nunc-Immuno   Poly-Sorp   für VHS und IHN
                              Maxi-Sorp   für IPN

Virus   VHS   Riems: Fi13   IHN -Typ1

Roti®-Block (10x Konzentrat) Carl Roth GmbH, Karlsruhe   (1:10 in Aqua dest.)

Waschpuffer   PBS-Tween 20   (0,5ml Tween/1l Aqua dest.)

Carbonatpuffer   3g NaHCO3/1l Aqua dest. mit Na2CO3 auf **pH 8,6**

Anti-Forellen-IgM von der Maus: mAk 4c10 (Eigenproduktion FLI)

Anti-Maus-Ig-OPD Konjugat   Pierce (Ziege)
                             Sigma (Kaninchen)

σ-Phenylendiamine Tablets (4mg)   Sigma-Aldrich

Phosphat-Citrat-Puffer **(pH 5)**
    A Posphat   0,2M Na2HPO4x 2H2O   (3,56g/100ml Aqua dest.)
    B Citrat   0,1M Zitronensäure   (2,1g/100ml Aqua dest.)

    A ca. 10,28ml mit **B** ca. 9,72ml zusammen geben, davon 10ml/1Tab. OPD

Wasserstoffperoxid (30%)

Schwefelsäure (4N)

Indirect capture ELISA according to Olesen and Jørgensen, DTU, Århus (Denmark)

1) Coating procedure
   a) Six ml coating buffer is necessary to coat 1 plate. Estimate 5ml extra for each following plate. Use 3 ml for ½ plate.
   b) Dilutions:
A. VHSV-ELISA: Protein-A purified rabbit anti-(F1-225) VHSV is diluted 1:750 with coating buffer.
B. IHNV-ELISA: Protein-A purified rabbit anti-IHNV (K33) diluted 1:1000 with coating buffer.
   c) 50 µl of diluted purified antibody is added to each well of the plate.
   d) Incubate the plate ON (over night) at 4°C in a humid chamber on an orbital shaker.

2) Virus antigen layer
   a) The ELISA-plate coated with Protein-A purified anti-VHSV or anti-IHNV is washed immediately after incubation.
   b) Virus (in breeding medium solution) is diluted 1:10 in PBS-T-BSA (approx. 3 ml is necessary for one plate). IHNV is diluted 1:5 in PBS-T-BSA (approx. 3 ml for one plate).
   c) 50 µl of diluted virus antigen is added only to row A-F. In other rows (C-H) 50 µl of dilution buffer (PBS-T-BSA) is added.
   d) Incubate the plate for 1h at 20°C in a humid chamber on an orbital shaker.
   e) The plate is washed immediately after incubation.

3) Blocking
   a) 100 µl of blocking buffer (PBS-T-BSA) is added to each well.
   b) Incubate the plate for 2h at 20°C in a humid chamber on an orbital shaker.
   c) The plate is washed immediately after incubation.

4) Incubation of the samples and controls
   a) Preparation of dilution plate: another 96-well plate is with 272 µl PBS-T-BSA in row A and E, all other wells are filled with 180 µl PBS-T-BSA. Add 8 µl of the tested serum to well A1 and E1, next tested serum to well A2 and E2 etc. After adding all sera in row A and E, mix the whole dilution well and transfer 60 µl into row B and F and mix again. Like that, transfer again 60 µl from row B and F into C and G and also 60 µl from row C and H.
   b) 50 µl of each dilution is transferred from the dilution plate to the washed and blocking ELISA-plate. Each dilution is transferred twice, i.e. column 1 from dilution plate is placed in column 1 and 2 of ELISA-plate, column 2 in 3 and

4 etc. In one ELISA-plate 10 samples and one positive and negative control can be incubated.

c) Incubate the plate ON at 4°C in a humid chamber on an orbital shaker.

d) The plate is washed immediately after incubation

1st layer	2nd layer	4rd layer	
α-VHSV	VHSV	A	Serum + PBS 1:40
		B	Serum + PBS 1:160
		C	Serum + PBS 1:640
		D	Serum + PBS 1:2560
	Buffer	E	Serum + PBS 1:40
		F	Serum + PBS 1:160
		G	Serum + PBS 1:640
		H	Serum + PBS 1:2560

6) <u>Incubation of the primary antibody</u>

a) MAb 4C10 (anti-rainbow trout IgM) is diluted 1:50 in PBS-T-BSA. MAb D_2 (anti rainbow trout IgM) is diluted 1:1000 in PBS-T-BSA. Use 6 ml of the dilution buffer with both antibodies inside for one plate and estimate 5 ml for each following plate.

b) Transfer 50 µl to each well.

c) Incubate the plate for 1h at 20°C in a humid chamber on an orbital shaker.

d) The plate is washed immediately after incubation.

7) <u>Incubation of the secondary conjugated antibody</u>

a) HPR-conjugated rabbit anti-mouse immunoglobulins are diluted 1:1000 in PBS-T-BSA. Use 6 ml for a whole plate and estimate 5 ml extra for each following plate.

b) Transfer 50 µl to each well.

c) Incubate the plate for 1h at 20°C in a humid chamber on a orbital shaker.

d) The plate is washed immediately after incubation.

8) <u>Development of ELISA</u>

a) Use ODP-tablets (Sigma) as the conjugate recommended by product instructions, 50µl each well.

9) <u>Stop color reaction</u>

a) Add 100 µl sulfuric acid (5N) to each well.

10) <u>Monitoring the absorbance</u>

a) Absorbance is measured spectrophotometrically at a wavelength of 492 nm in an ELISA reader.

Materials for the indirect capture ELISA

96-well microplates	Greiner Microplates F high binding (655061)

Coating Buffer (pH=9.6)	Na_2CO_3 .... 0,795 g
	$NaHCO_3$ .... 1,465 g
	Milli Q water .... 500 ml

PBS Stock Solution	$NaH_2PO_4 \cdot H_2O$ .... 8,63 g
(1:5)	$Na_2HPO_4 \cdot 12\ H_2O$ .... 67,00 g
	NaCl .... 211,90 g
	Milli Q water .... fill up to 5l

Procedure:
1. Add all salts to a 2l glass bottle and fill up 2l with Milli Q water.
2. Stir on a magnetic stirrer in a refrigerator at 4°C, if necessary overnight.
3. Transfer the solution to a 5l glass bottle and add 3l Mill Q water. Check pH for the diluted solution, e.g. 10 ml stock solution + 40 ml Milli Q water (i.e. a dilution of 1:5) should have a pH value of 7.2 ± 0.2. Do not adjust pH if values are outside these limits, but discard the batch.
4. Store in a refrigerator at 4°C. Allow to adjust to room temperature before diluting 1:5 with Milli Q water before use. Storage for 3 month.

PBS Washing Buffer	PBS Stock Solution .... 200 ml
	Milli Q water .... 800 ml
	Tween 20 .... 2,4 ml

PBS-T-BSA	PBS Washing Buffer plus 1%BSA

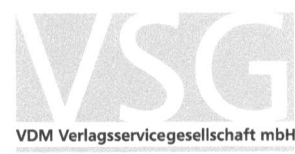

VDM Verlagsservicegesellschaft mbH

Die VDM Verlagsservicegesellschaft sucht für wissenschaftliche Verlage abgeschlossene und herausragende

Dissertationen, Habilitationen, Diplomarbeiten, Master Theses, Magisterarbeiten usw.

für die kostenlose Publikation als Fachbuch.

Sie verfügen über eine Arbeit, die hohen inhaltlichen und formalen Ansprüchen genügt, und haben Interesse an einer honorarvergüteten Publikation?

Dann senden Sie bitte erste Informationen über sich und Ihre Arbeit per Email an *info@vdm-vsg.de*.

Sie erhalten kurzfristig unser Feedback!

VDM Verlagsservicegesellschaft mbH
Dudweiler Landstr. 99
D - 66123 Saarbrücken
www.vdm-vsg.de

Telefon +49 681 3720 174
Fax   +49 681 3720 1749

Die VDM Verlagsservicegesellschaft mbH vertritt

 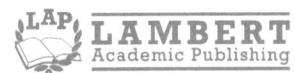 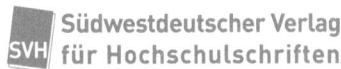

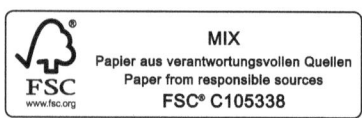

Printed by Books on Demand GmbH, Norderstedt / Germany